TAKE
CONTROL
OF YOUR
CANCER
RISK

TAKE CONTROL
OF YOUR
CANCER
RISK

JOHN WHYTE, MD, MPH

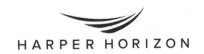

HARPER HORIZON

ISBN 978-0-7852-4041-9 (eBook)
ISBN 978-0-7852-4040-2 (HC)

Library of Congress Control Number: 2021931680

Printed in the United States of America
21 22 23 24 25 LSC 10 9 8 7 6 5 4 3 2 1

TO ALISA

May everyone be as fortunate as
we have been to find a life partner.

TO LUKE AND JACK

You give me purpose in life.

An ounce of PREVENTION

is worth a pound of CURE.

—BENJAMIN FRANKLIN

CONTENTS

CHAPTER NINE

INTRODUCTION

"YOU HAVE CANCER." The three scariest words to hear.

If you or a loved one has been diagnosed with a condition such as heart disease or diabetes, you might have thought, *Well, at least it's not cancer.* We still dread a cancer diagnosis. That's justified because, despite a war on cancer launched nearly fifty years ago, cancer remains a leading cause of death. While it's true that we have witnessed a tremendous explosion of new drugs and treatments that target specific cancer cells, treatment is no walk in the park. It may cure you, but it may also decrease your quality of life and shorten it.

The biggest myth I hear regarding cancer is that it's mostly caused by genetics. That is so wrong! Although genetics plays a role in whether you'll develop cancer, most experts agree it accounts for less than 20 percent of cancer. The little-known truth is that lifestyle and the environment play the major roles. Let me phrase that another way: what you eat, how you exercise, how much you sleep, your outlook on life, where you live, and how you live mostly determines whether you get cancer.

We need a mindset change from "I hope I don't get cancer" to "How I can prevent cancer?"

Believe it not, you have the power to reduce your risk of many cancers. We have more data now than ever before showing what you can do—what you need to do—to prevent a cancer diagnosis.

I want you to think about cancer in the same way you do heart disease or stroke. Even if your parents had a heart attack, you don't think you're automatically destined to the same fate. Rather, I bet you try to keep your weight under control, watch your blood pressure and cholesterol level, and might even try to increase your physical activity. You're playing a proactive role in whether you'll have a heart attack or become debilitated from a stroke. The approach to cancer should be the same because your decisions play a major role in your risk of being diagnosed with cancer. Of course, nothing is 100 percent effective, but science can now show you how to reduce your personal risk.

Also, I want to highlight at least one important difference with cancer. Unlike with heart attacks or stroke, with cancer, you don't often get a second chance to make those lifestyle changes. That's why it is so important for you to understand the power you have in creating your personal cancer prevention program.

Today, medical professionals recognize cancer as not one disease but more a collection of different diseases. And we know with good certainty what strategies can help decrease the risk for different types of cancer. It's not the same exact recommendations for breast cancer as for colon cancer or even for ovarian cancer or prostate cancer. There are similarities, but it's not a one-size-fits-all approach.

Even when you practice prevention, you still need to know how to recognize cancer signs and symptoms. Just because you don't smoke doesn't mean you won't get lung cancer. How do you know when a chronic cough is a lingering viral illness versus something more serious? When should you be concerned about unintentional weight loss in yourself or a loved one? I'll give you answers to these questions, and much more.

One important proactive strategy for cancer prevention is screenings. However, the screening process can be confusing. When should you get screened, and for what cancers? Which test is best? Too many patients have told me they don't need to get mammography or colonoscopy because "it doesn't run in their family" or "I'm fine. I don't have any symptoms." That should never be your reasoning. To help prevent cancer, it's critical to be screened for the different types. And currently, it seems that we need to be screening for some cancers much earlier than we previously thought.

You're also likely aware of other factors that contribute to minimizing risk for different cancer types, including but not limited to diet, exercise, sleep, and attitude. For instance, you may know that it's good to eat a "healthy" diet, but what does that really mean? With exercise, does it matter what type you do, or is any increase in movement sufficient? How do you know if you're getting too much or too little sleep? Can a positive attitude reduce your cancer risk?

So, what exactly do you do? How do you empower yourself to make the right decisions? It can be hard to know where to begin, and the cacophony of different "experts" espousing often conflicting advice can be confusing. Some of it is hype; some of it is shameless marketing; and some of it is excellent information based on the latest science. That's why it's important to rely on credible, trustworthy sources. It is your body and your life—and you deserve the best information, which will lead to better health.

That's where this book comes into play. *Take Control of Your Cancer Risk* is your essential guide to the most up-to-date information, backed by science. It distills the data and information to the most relevant, salient points, so you can understand and implement.

Let's get started.

TAKE
CONTROL
OF YOUR
CANCER
RISK

CHAPTER ONE

Can Cancer Really Be Prevented?

TRUE OR FALSE?

1. Cancer rates have been decreasing in the last five years.
2. Women are more likely to die from cancer than men.
3. Cancer is the number one cause of death among Americans.
4. Blacks are diagnosed with cancer more often than whites.
5. Brushing your teeth can help prevent cancer.

(Answers at end of chapter)

EVERY TIME I SEE MY patient "Joe," I talk to him about his weight and his smoking—and every time, he shrugs me off. His typical response sounds something like this: "Dr. Whyte, I know people who did everything right. They never smoked, didn't drink, exercised every day, and they still got cancer. I'm not stopping what I enjoy."

He's right. Some people seem to do everything right but still get cancer. And just like Joe, we might take that to mean that we can't do anything to prevent cancer, so why waste our time trying.

I understand why people might think this way—sometimes cancer does seem random, striking without reason. We may think we are powerless to prevent cancer because, even though there are more treatments for cancer than ever before, many of us still see cancer as a death sentence. Tell someone you've got cancer—no matter what kind or what stage—and they will probably immediately be sad and worried about your longevity. Some people are so afraid of cancer, they won't even call it by name. Even when you might have suspicious symptoms, you might not want to find out—due to the fear of a cancer diagnosis. You've heard of "FOMO"—fear of missing out. But for cancer—there's "FOFO"—fear of finding out. Many cancers are diagnosed late because patients just don't want to have to deal with a cancer diagnosis, so they ignore symptoms, or attribute them to some other condition. If we think of cancer as a disease striking at random, it's no wonder that many of us assume that we can't prevent it, or at least reduce our chances of getting it.

But cancer is not unstoppable or completely random.

In fact, we've been making some headway. Cancer rates have been falling for the past twenty-five years—down nearly 30 percent during this time. Preventive measures such as quitting smoking and wearing sunscreen help explain this decline. We've also developed sophisticated technologies that have improved screening, and we have made huge advances in treatment. It's a story of success—or partial success.

Sadly, there's also bad news. I don't want you to think we have won the war against cancer just yet. Far from it! Each year, more than 1.7 million new cases of cancer are diagnosed and more than 600,000 people die from it (see Figure 1). That's each year. Every year. In fact, cancer is overtaking heart disease as the leading cause of death in the US. Just as we focus on preventing heart attacks, we need to focus on preventing cancer. We all have a general awareness of cancer; most of us know someone who has suffered from it—a friend or loved one. Yet, we don't act to prevent it as we do with diabetes, heart attacks, and strokes.

One reason we don't approach cancer prevention as we do other diseases is that many of us wrongly believe that our genes primarily determine whether we will get cancer. This is not true! Genetics does play a part, but not as much as people think. Data suggests that less than 20 percent of cancers are inherited through our genes– that leaves a lot of room for prevention!

Some people believe that if they get cancer, they will undergo treatment and conquer their disease. Some do, but unfortunately many do not. Despite the innovations we have in *treatments*, I want you to know about any means we have to *prevent* cancer and incorporate them in my life. Let's not try to treat our way out of cancer; let's prevent it. I'm not going to wait for a cure that may never come or rely on therapies that may not improve my quality of life. I hope you feel the same.

What Does Prevention Mean When It Comes to Cancer?

Experts agree that around 70 percent of cancer may be prevented by reducing risk factors and undergoing adequate

NEW CANCER CASES BY SITE (YEARLY)

MALE

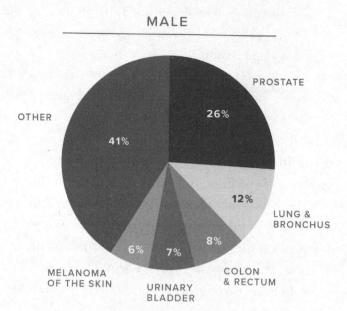

FEMALE

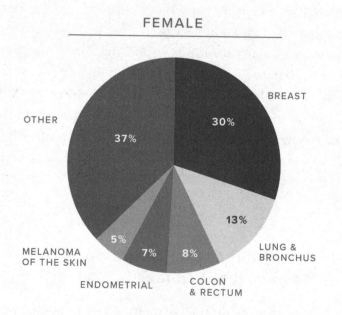

Figure 1

screening. This doesn't mean that cancer is completely preventable, but you can certainly improve your chances.

If you want to do all you can to prevent cancer, it's important to know what increases your risk. Some of those risks you can eliminate, and some you can't. Awareness is the first step. I want you to be empowered with the knowledge that will allow you to take control.

First, let's talk about risk in a broad sense, looking at how cancer affects the population. Think about it this way—most Americans have a 1 in 3 chance of getting cancer in their lifetime. Some people have greater risk than others. Women are diagnosed with cancer more often than men. In terms of dying from cancer, your risk is 1 in 5. If you are Black or Hispanic, you are less likely to be diagnosed with cancer (see Figure 2). But once you are

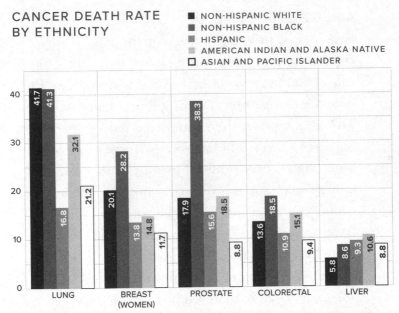

CANCER DEATH RATE BY ETHNICITY

- NON-HISPANIC WHITE
- NON-HISPANIC BLACK
- HISPANIC
- AMERICAN INDIAN AND ALASKA NATIVE
- ASIAN AND PACIFIC ISLANDER

LUNG: 41.7, 41.3, 16.8, 32.1, 21.2
BREAST (WOMEN): 20.1, 28.2, 13.8, 14.8, 11.7
PROSTATE: 17.9, 38.3, 15.6, 18.5, 8.8
COLORECTAL: 13.6, 18.5, 10.9, 15.1, 9.4
LIVER: 5.8, 8.6, 9.3, 10.6, 8.8

AVERAGE ANNUAL DEATH RATE PER 100,000 US STANDARD POPULATION (2014–2018)

Figure 2

diagnosed, your risk of dying from it is much higher than whites. Why? Cancer is often diagnosed much later in minority populations, so it is further along by the time it's discovered. Minorities also have more risk factors and less access to cancer treatments—a bad combination. Historically, people of color have not had equal access to treatment for cancer care, especially for breast, prostate, and colorectal cancer—and inequality persists.

That's the broad view of risk—and it can be helpful to keep in mind—but your personal risk is mostly determined by a combination of individual risk factors. The following list has some things you can change, and some you can't.

What Puts You at Risk?

- **Age.** We used to think cancer was primarily a disease related to aging, but it's much more complicated than that. How old you are does play a big role in whether you get cancer, and it's important to be aware of what cancers typically occur at what age. The older you are, the greater your risk of developing some cancers will be, because some cancers require many years to develop. But cancer doesn't only affect people who are over fifty. About 30 percent of cancer occurs in people younger than that. If you are a woman between twenty and fifty, you are more likely to be diagnosed with and die of cancer than men of the same age. Knowing how age might affect your risk can help you be more alert to cancer signs and symptoms.

- **Tobacco.** Approximately 16 percent of the population smokes. That's much better than in previous years, but it still represents tens of millions of people. If you smoke, you increase your risk of cancer dramatically. Please remember that secondhand smoke is deadly as well. If you are exposed to secondhand smoke at work or at home, your risk of lung cancer increases by a third. Don't think that smoking only affects your lungs. It also increases the chance of cancer of the esophagus, liver, pancreas, stomach, cervix, colon, rectum, and blood.

- **Obesity.** Carrying excess weight multiplies your risks. Cancers are decreasing, but not the ones associated with being overweight (gallbladder, stomach, pancreas, thyroid, liver, colon, ovarian). These are actually increasing.

- **Diet.** What you eat and how much plays an important role in determining your personal cancer risk. Highly processed foods and red meat, for example, increase your risk of cancer. Same holds true if you rarely eat fruits and vegetables, or struggle to include whole grains.

- **Alcohol.** Although there has been conflicting data, most data points to increased risk of some cancers (breast, colon, and esophageal cancer, for example) if your alcohol consumption is more than moderate. Moderate is defined as no more than one drink per day for women, two drinks per men, on five days of the week. You don't get to average consumption over the course of the week. It's the daily amount that affects risk.

- **Physical inactivity.** The less active you are, the greater your risk of cancer. This is an additional risk, separate from obesity. Even if you are skinny or at a healthy weight, if you don't exercise, your odds of getting cancer still go up.

- **Diabetes.** We know that type 2 diabetes is related to poor diet and physical inactivity leading to obesity, which are, in themselves, risk factors. But type 2 diabetes itself may be an independent risk factor for cancer. We still need to do more research, but poor glucose control and insulin resistance seems to increase your cancer risk.

- **UV radiation.** There's simply no such thing as a healthy tan. Too much sun increases your risk of skin cancer, especially basal cell and squamous cell cancers. I know people are focused on vitamin D nowadays and strive to get some sun exposure, but lack of protection against the sun's harmful rays causes cell damage that can accumulate over years. It's still not clear to me why people use tanning salons and tanning devices when the risk of cancer is well documented. Sunscreen, lip balm, sunglasses, and wide-brim hats need to be your friend!

- **Environmental pollution.** Polluted air and water and soil contaminated by carcinogenic chemicals can increase your cancer risk. We know its impact on asthma so it should not be surprising that pollution can impact your overall immunity. We have all seen those news stories in which several people in a community develop the same type of cancer living near a nuclear power plant or polluted water supply. These are not coincidences. Pollution can harm your cells, resulting in mutations that increase cancer risk.

- **Occupational exposure.** The most infamous example has been asbestos, which causes cancer of the lung and other organs (mesothelioma). People who work around heavy metals (nickel, lead, cadmium, for example) or in coal mining, woodworking, or rubber making are at increased risk. Vinyl chloride, a chemical involved with plastic, also has been shown to increase risk. Here's a problem when it comes to these exposures: don't assume your employer will tell you about possible cancer risks associated with your job. You need to ask, and sometimes do your own research. The most common mode of transmission is through inhalation and the skin. Lung, bladder, and non-Hodgkin's lymphoma have been the cancers most commonly associated with occupational exposures. Keep in mind that, if you are outside most of the day doing your job, UV radiation from sun exposure can also be considered an occupational exposure.

- **Infections.** Infections pose a greater risk in developing countries but still cause almost 10 percent of all cancers in the United States and Canada. Viruses are the main culprit, but bacteria and parasites are also implicated. HPV, HIV, hepatitis B and C, H pylori, schistosomiasis, herpes, and Epstein-Barr are the typical infections associated with cancer. They don't automatically lead to cancer, but we should try to prevent these infections as well as diagnosing and treating them. In doing so, we will decrease the rates of many cancers, especially worldwide.

- **Poor dental health.** People with severe gum disease have nearly a 25 percent increased risk in developing cancer compared to those with no gum disease. Oral health and cancer are connected in ways we are just beginning to understand. Bacteria in our mouth as well as inflammation from poor oral hygiene are probably the causes. Nobody really likes to floss, but healthy mouths leads to healthy bodies. So, brush your teeth! And floss too!

- **Disability.** People with a chronic disability are at increased risk. This may not seem to make sense when you first look at it, but part of the risk may be the lifestyle challenges that people with disabilities face. It may also be related to potentially decreased immunity related to disability. Research does show increases in prostate, colorectal, ovarian, and non-Hodgkin's lymphoma in persons with disabilities that are associated with movement difficulties. Given that roughly 15 percent of the population may have a disability, this is an association we need to recognize and address. We know that people with disabilities don't always receive comprehensive cancer care when they are diagnosed, so it's all the more important to be aware that many are at increased risk. Patients with disabilities may need more cancer screening, and we may need to be more alert for subtle cancer symptoms. We also should develop strategies to make sure people with disabilities can benefit from exercise and address mental health issues that can lead to tobacco and alcohol use.

- **Medications.** Every so often, we hear about medications that increase cancer risk. Your pharmacist might contact you about a recall of a drug you are taking, especially given the US Food and Drug Administration's increased inspection of drug manufacturing and enhanced drug quality standards. Sometimes the danger comes from contaminants in the medication, such as N-Nitrosodimethylamine (NDMA). Other times it's due to the medication's effect on our bodies. For example, hydrochlorothiazide, a diuretic often used to treat high blood pressure, increases sensitivity to light. Some antibiotics and antifungals do also, although for a shorter period of time. The photosensitivity may slightly increase risks for certain skin cancers. The long-term use of hormone replacement therapy (particularly the long-term use of estrogen without any countering progesterone) has been associated with increased rates of some cancers. Don't stop taking a drug without talking to your doctor—but you might need to switch to a different drug, or increase screening.

- **Hidradenitis suppurativa.** This is a skin condition that often forms lumps—sometimes with pus— under the skin, often the armpit or the groin. A recent study conducted in Korea showed increase in cancer rates with greater risk if you have moderate to severe condition. The risk is still low, and is related to invasive cancers.

- **Gout.** If you have a history of gout, your risk for lung cancer, urological cancer, and digestive cancer is much higher than someone who has never had gout. Gout's high cell turnover and inflammation, as well as high serum uric acid, seem to play a role in the potential growth of tumor cells. It is important that you try to keep your gout under control through diet and medication. If you have frequent gout attacks, it could be a warning sign, and you need to take note. You might need to get screened more often for cancer than you typically might if you didn't have frequent gout attacks.

- **Autoimmune disease.** You can't control whether you develop an autoimmune disease like ulcerative colitis, Crohn's, lupus, rheumatoid arthritis, or multiple sclerosis. But you do need to know that you are at increased risk for certain cancers such as colorectal disease, brain, or lung cancer depending on your underlying condition. The disease might induce your body to attack normal cells, and some of the treatments used to treat your condition may impair your body's ability to fight growing tumors.

- **X-rays.** Getting dental X-rays, chest X-rays, and CT scans can be important diagnostic tools, but too much radiation can increase the risks of some cancers, including bone, thyroid, and breast. In general, medical X-rays use low amounts of radiation so the risk is minimal. However, the more X-rays and scans you have, the more the risk increases given the amount of total radiation. Even if you only get a few X-rays each year, be sure to wear a lead blanket and not get too many tests in a short period of time.

These risks can be additive—meaning if you have more than one, they add up in determining your overall risk.

What Does Not Increase Risk

Since we are discussing what increases risk, let's also discuss a few things that do *not* elevate risk—despite what you might read and hear from some people. Cell phones and power lines do not increase cancer risk. Nor do antiperspirants or deodorants. No data suggests that fluoride in toothpaste or drinking water causes cancer. Sugar does not cause cancer to grow, and neither do any artificial sweeteners on the market show evidence of increased cancer risk.

What about those old dental fillings? No need to get them replaced. The amount of mercury is actually small, and it's often mixed with traces of other metals. There's no link between these fillings and cancer.

Recent data shows that fertility drugs used to assist pregnancy do not seem to increase cancer risk. Using a microwave does not increase rates of cancer. Hair dyes have been linked to cancer—particularly bladder cancer—but the risk seems concentrated in those, such as barbers and hair stylists, who may be exposed to dye throughout the day. You're not at risk if you simply dye your hair a few times a year.

There's also no data that shows plastic water bottles increase your chances of getting cancer. Same thing for power lines—the electrical energy does not change your cells.

Lack of Awareness

How many of these risk factors were you aware of? Most people are unaware or misinformed about their risks of getting cancer. I'm glad you are reading this book so you can learn what puts you at increased risk of getting cancer and take action.

In a recent survey, the American Society of Clinical Oncology asked people what they know about cancer. The results were fascinating. For example, only 30 percent polled knew that obesity and alcohol are risk factors for cancer. Nearly 80 percent were unaware of the role of viruses in increasing cancer risk.

You might be like some of my patients who tell me, "Doc, I don't know what to believe anymore. Some days, it seems like everything causes cancer." I appreciate that because it provides an opportunity to separate fact from fiction. Unfortunately, less than a quarter of adults report talking to a doctor about their cancer risk, and even fewer ask what they can do to reduce it. Honestly, I'm frustrated by the many doctors who don't adequately discuss your risk or what modifications you can make to reduce it. Even cancer specialists rarely tell their patients what they can do to improve their overall health or reduce cancer recurrence. As a result, two-thirds of consumers are unsure about which sources to trust for information on what causes cancer. It can be confusing. The media can make it even more difficult, since they only give highlights of studies, with very little detail. It can be hard to figure out based on different reports when you personally should get a mammogram or whether you should be drinking more than two cups of coffee a day. As you strive to take control of your cancer risk, it's important to get credible information from trusted sources.

Awareness of risk factors is the first step. The second step is action. By taking steps to manage your risk factors, you may be able to reduce your risk, and possibly prevent cancer. No one is promising that you can completely control whether you get cancer, but you can control how well you manage your risk factors. Again, this is where we need to start treating cancer like a preventable disease. We all know that by making lifestyle changes we can reduce risk of heart disease and diabetes. The same is true for cancer. Yet, only one in four people says they incorporate cancer prevention into their daily life.

Let's change that.

I know that making lifestyle changes can be difficult. Unhealthy habits are hard to break! But preventing cancer is worth the effort. Yes, we do have more effective cancer treatments than ever before. But even with the innovations, treatments have side effects, some serious, and success is not guaranteed. Why go through all that if you can avoid it? And don't automatically assume you will get the best care if you get cancer. Unfortunately, not everybody will receive equal treatment.

By reading the next few chapters, you will learn what you need to do to make cancer prevention a part of your life. You might be able to avoid the pain and suffering that often comes with a cancer diagnosis. Let me help teach you ways to reduce your odds of getting cancer, so you can make them part of your life.

Please don't have the attitude that you will wait for a cure. I hope we will find a cure for cancer one day. But don't be misled into thinking a cure is the only way we can ever be free of cancer. A good friend who is a cancer doctor said to me several years ago: "Let's hope for a cure, John, but plan to be cancer-free through real prevention." Lifestyle changes are worth your time. They may not be "glitzy" or have the "wow-effect" of the latest drugs, but making lifestyle changes works!

The good news is, preventive steps are simple (notice I did not say "easy"!), and if you start making changes, even just one at a time, you can lower your risk of developing cancer. Although no cancer is 100 percent preventable, you do have control over many risk factors. In the next eight chapters, you will be empowered to advocate for yourself and to create your personal cancer prevention program. You can take control of your cancer risk.

Summary

Despite advances in treatment, cancer remains a leading cause of death. The types of cancer that have increased over the past few years have changed; many of them are caused by things that we have control over: diet, alcohol and tobacco use, lack of exercise, and poor sleeping habits.

Genetics plays a small part in whether you get cancer. This means you can play an important role in reducing your odds of a cancer diagnosis. Start thinking about cancer as something you can help prevent. Learn the risk factors and take action!

ANSWERS

1. **TRUE**—Cancer rates overall have been decreasing. However, some cancers are increasing among some groups. That's why it is so important to develop your personal cancer prevention program.

2. **FALSE**—Women are less likely to die from cancer than men.

3. **FALSE**—Cancer is not the number one cause of death but continues to kill many Americans each year.

4. **FALSE**—Blacks are diagnosed with cancer less frequently than whites, but a greater percentage of those diagnosed with cancer die.

5. **TRUE**—Maintaining good oral health can reduce your risk of cancer.

CHAPTER TWO

What's My Personal Risk for Cancer?

TRUE OR FALSE?

1. Doctors can accurately predict your cancer risk.
2. If you're Black or Hispanic, it's harder to estimate your chances of developing skin cancer.
3. Online risk calculators don't apply to people with genetic mutations.
4. Cancer risk changes as you get older.
5. Even if you develop cancer, your chances of being cured are good.

(Answers at end of chapter)

IF YOU WERE DRIVING ON a steep, winding cliffside road at night, you'd want to have a good view of how close you were to the edge, right? You'd probably prefer to have a very wide shoulder—and a sturdy guardrail—between you and that drop-off. But what if you didn't? What if the edge of that road was right at the edge of the cliff? I bet you'd be very glad that you could see where the edge is exactly (thank goodness for headlights!); and that you would be paying close attention to that edge—being very careful that you keep your car from drifting too far toward it and possibly going over.

Of course, you have more control over how close you are to the cliff edge (and not all cancers are as deadly as driving off a cliff). You don't have as much control over avoiding cancer, but I give this dramatic example to emphasize how important it is to get a clear understanding of your cancer risk. Just as you would want to know the distance between your car and that cliff, wouldn't you want to understand how close you might be to cancer?

In the last chapter, we surveyed the risk factors for cancer. There are a lot of them. What's exciting is that we can now get specific and look at your own personal risk!

We already do this for heart disease, diabetes, and stroke. Do you know your risk for a heart attack? How likely are you to have a stroke? If you give me a few data points, I can tell you your ten-year or five-year risk. This information helps us manage and optimize your health, especially as it relates to lifestyle changes and medicines.

Heart doctors have always been good about collecting data that helps estimate your risk. And that's really what you care about, isn't it? You want to know your chances of suffering a heart attack or a stroke. Of course, these calculators aren't 100 percent accurate, but they do provide useful information that can help you take control to prevent or delay a heart attack or stroke. They also give your doctor insight to help maximize your personal care. By getting an idea how far away you are from the "cliff," you and your doctor can create a plan to course correct.

I routinely calculate heart disease risk for my patients—and myself! It helps make risk more "real" when you see your own numbers. In the past we didn't have the medical tools to make these calculations, but now we do.

We need the same approach for cancer. It's a bit more challenging, since cancer represents a range of diseases, not just one, like heart disease or diabetes. I can't tell you your risk for "cancer," but instead I might be able to tell you your personal risk for breast cancer or colon cancer or lung cancer.

Because cancer has always seemed mysterious to many people, it often surprises them that we have calculators for cancer risk. Over the last few years, however, we have learned the various risk factors for different types of cancer, and we've put them in a "calculator" to help predict your personal risk. It's not absolute—meaning, a low score is no guarantee you won't get the disease in the next few years, or if it's high, that you need to get your affairs in order.

Rather, this information empowers you to become involved in your own health care. That's critical. I'm a big fan of giving people information. After all, information is power. It's important that you have as much information as you can, and your chance of getting cancer is one of the things you need to know.

Numerous online risk calculators exist to provide your personalized risk for different types of cancers. Some were originally designed for physicians to help assess their patients, but nowadays you can input the data and do the calculation yourself. The key is to review the results with your physician. Patients are increasingly becoming partners with their doctor to help decide their care. Getting some basic information will be helpful to both of you and may increase your motivation to take control of your cancer risk. Don't just calculate your risk and then forget about it. Rather, use the opportunity to take control.

Obesity Calculator

You will find that many cancer risk calculators include a question about your height and weight to determine whether you are overweight or obese. Many people aren't realistic about how many excess pounds they carry, so it's good to get the numbers so you and your doctor can decide what you need to do. Although there has been some controversy about body-mass index, it's still one of the best measures we have. And yes, it doesn't account for how much of that mass is muscle, but let's be honest—most of us aren't muscular.

BMI requires a bit of math; it is calculated by dividing weight by height. Thankfully, there are lots of different calculators online to do the thinking for you—all you have to do is put in your height and weight and the calculator tells you if you are overweight, a healthy weight, or underweight. Please also make sure you are measuring your height accurately. I find that people simply use a height that they've been saying since they were twenty. When was the last time you had your height measured? Lots of times you are simply asked how tall you are. Get a measurement every year because we do start shrinking when we're in our thirties; over time, we can become an inch or even two inches shorter. Combine that with the fact that most of us gain weight as we get older and you might be in for a surprise when you do your BMI calculation.

Another good measure when it comes to obesity is waist circumference. We know that belly fat is metabolically active—it secretes hormones and chemicals that cause inflammation throughout our body. This inflammation can impact your cancer risk, so the size of your waist provides useful information as you develop your personal cancer prevention program. So, how do you measure it?

1. Start at the top of your hip bone, then bring the tape measure all the way around your body, level with your belly button.
2. Make sure it's not too tight and that it's straight, even at the back. Don't hold your breath while measuring. There's no need to impress anyone! Whenever I measure a patient's waist, they invariably "suck it in." Please don't do that. We need accurate information.
3. Check the number on the tape measure right after you exhale.

For your best health, your waist should be less than forty inches around for men, and less than thirty-five inches for women (see Figure 3).

WAIST CIRCUMFERENCE

HEALTH RISK	FEMALES	MALES
NORMAL	<35 IN (<88 CM)	<40 IN (<102 CM)
INCREASED	>35 IN (>88 CM)	>40 IN (>102 CM)

Figure 3

Remember: we can't spot-reduce fat in isolated areas of the body. That's why it's a good idea to measure the waist. It is a good reflection of the amount of fat in your body. And don't cheat—for men reading, it's not the waist size of your pants!

Risk Calculators

There isn't a well-validated risk calculator for every type of cancer. At least, not yet. As you plan to reduce your risk of specific cancers, consider checking out the risk calculators for the following cancers: skin, colon, prostate, breast, lung.

Skin Cancer

This calculator, created by the National Cancer Institute (NCI), helps assess your five-year risk of developing melanoma, the most serious form of skin cancer.

https://mrisktool.cancer.gov/calculator.html

This tool assesses the following risk criteria:

- Race
- Age
- Gender
- Complexion (light, medium, dark)
- Geographic location (northern, central, southern, for example)
- History of blistering sunburns

- Presence of moles larger than five millimeters on the back (roughly half the size of a pencil eraser); Fewer than two, or two or more?
- Presence of moles less than five millimeters on the back (fewer than seven; seven to sixteen; or more than seventeen)
- Amount of freckling on back and shoulders (is it absent, mild, moderate, severe?)
- Sun damage on shoulders

Please note that this calculator cannot be used for everyone. It mostly applies to non-Hispanic whites, between the ages of twenty and seventy. This model has not been tested in large populations and may not be accurate if you are Black or Hispanic. Unfortunately, the field of dermatology has not devoted equal resources to studying skin cancer in people of color. This risk calculator also doesn't apply if you have had melanoma or other skin cancers, or a family history of melanoma.

Colorectal Cancer

This risk calculator is also designed by the NCI. Designed for people between the ages of forty-five and eighty-five, the calculator estimates your personal five-year risk of getting colorectal cancer, as well as your lifetime risk. A nice component of this tool is that it compares your personal risk based on your answers to the average risk. This calculator doesn't apply to people with genetic mutations since their risk is higher than average.

https://ccrisktool.cancer.gov/

You will need to input the following:

- Age
- Sex
- Race/Ethnicity
- Height
- Weight
- Number of servings of vegetables or leafy green salads consumed per week
- Amount of moderate and vigorous physical activity you do per week and for how many months
- Normal or abnormal colonoscopy in the past ten years
- Presence of polyps on past colonoscopies
- Use of medications containing aspirin, or non-steroidal anti-inflammatories (NSAIDS)
- Family history of colon or rectal cancer
- Whether you ever smoked one hundred or more cigarettes in your lifetime

Prostate Cancer

If you are a man between fifty-five and seventy-four years of age, and want to know your risk, you might want to use the risk calculator designed by scientists at the Prostate Cancer Research Foundation. You can calculate your personal risk with or without a PSA level.

http://www.prostatecancer-riskcalculator.com/seven -prostate-cancer-risk-calculators

There's a couple of different calculators on this page and you can choose based on whether you already have a PSA level. I like these calculators because they don't just ask about family history, but also query you with key questions on symptoms. For instance, how many times you get up at night to urinate is a factor in determining your risk, as well as if you have the sensation of not being able to fully empty your bladder. Whether you have to urinate less than two hours after you previously did so is also a factor. Your results are presented on a chart that shows if you are below average, average, or above average. This information can help lead a discussion with your doctor.

Breast Cancer

The risk calculator, also developed by NCI, helps estimate your risk of developing invasive breast cancer over the next five years and up to age ninety. Like several of the other calculators, it only applies to women of average risk between ages thirty-five to eighty-five.

https://bcrisktool.cancer.gov/

The tool takes into consideration the following criteria:

- Age at first menstrual period
- Race/Ethnicity
- How old you were when you first gave birth (if you have children)
- History of breast cancer in any first-degree relative
- Past biopsy results

It is important to remember this tool doesn't apply to you if you have any genetic mutations (such as BRCA1 or

BRCA2). It also doesn't apply if you have a previous history of invasive or in situ breast cancer. If you are a Black or Hispanic woman, take note. The tool does state that it may underestimate risk in Black women with previous biopsies and Hispanic women born outside the United States. Because data on American Indian/Alaska Native women is limited, their risk estimates are partly based on data for white women and may be inaccurate.

This calculator gives your personal five-year risk of developing breast cancer and compares it to average risk. Based on your current answers, it also calculates your personal lifetime risk and compares it to average lifetime risk. You might find these numbers helpful in deciding how you will take control of your risk. For instance, some research suggests that women at high-risk (five-year risk > 3 percent) may benefit from medications such as tamoxifen, raloxifene, anastrozole, or exemestane that are used to reduce risk of invasive estrogen-receptor positive breast cancer.

Lung Cancer

If you or a loved one is a smoker, you might want to use this tool designed by the NCI to help determine five-year risk of developing lung cancer as well as five-year risk of dying from lung cancer.

analysistools.cancer.gov/lungCancerRiskAssessment/#/

As you might expect, smoking status is a key component of the calculator. It also includes:

• Current or former smoker

- Number of packs per day multiplied by number of years
- Age
- Gender
- Race/Ethnicity
- Height
- Weight
- Body mass index
- Highest level of education
- History of lung disease (for example, COPD, emphysema, chronic bronchitis)
- Family history of lung disease

Although lung cancer can occur in nonsmokers, this tool only applies to smokers or former smokers.

You Have a Risk Score. Now What?

Now that you have a risk score, what does it mean, and what do you do with it? Many of you will have very low numbers. Some of you might have a number that's higher than you expected. What can you do about it? What should you do about it?

These numbers are estimates and they can be confusing. Decimals and percentage points with zeros can be maddening! Many of us aren't good at math! What does .01 percent really mean? Would it be better if it said your chances are 1 in 10,000? What about 1 in 1,000? Does it feel the same? Or does one make you more concerned than the other? The way information is presented can have an impact. We also all have different reference points. A rate of 1 in 10,000 may seem low to you but high to your sister or father. How does it compare to other health conditions or life events? Having some type of comparison is helpful as you make decisions that impact your risk of getting cancer. Too often in life, we focus on rare events such as winning the Powerball lottery (1 in 300 million) or the odds of getting struck by lightning (1 in 200,000). We wear our seat belts and drive slowly when it's icy because we don't want to be involved in a car accident, where the risk is roughly 1 in 100. Yet, the overall risk of getting cancer is 1 in 3 and dying from cancer is 1 in 7 (see Figure 4). Let's keep that in perspective as you develop an action plan to reduce your cancer risk.

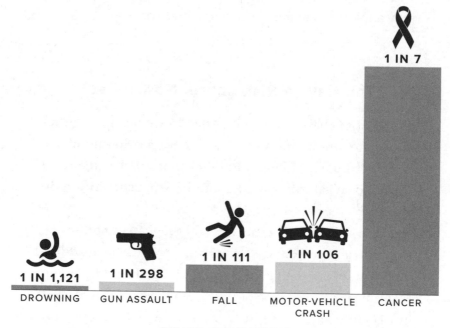

1 IN 7

1 IN 1,121   1 IN 298   1 IN 111   1 IN 106

DROWNING   GUN ASSAULT   FALL   MOTOR-VEHICLE CRASH   CANCER

ODDS OF DEATH

Figure 4

Some risk calculators categorize risk as low, moderate, or high to give some comparison to the average person. This can be helpful, but keep in mind that even low percentages can impact your overall health and risk of cancer. Even if your risk is "low," that doesn't mean you don't have to worry about screening tests or that you don't need to focus on eating healthy, getting restorative sleep, and exercising. Remember, your weight is a component in many of these calculators, and when that changes along with age, your risk might change too. So, your risk today might be different than it will be in five or ten years. Many of the behaviors that impact risk may take years or even decades to show their harmful effect. The good news is that you can control many of them.

If your risk is high, it's critical that you take actions to lower your risk. I would recommend making an appointment with your doctor to discuss your results and the steps you need to take to protect yourself. Some might be related to lifestyle change and others might mean more frequent screenings. This risk information also helps you to be more attuned to signs and symptoms of specific cancers. Understanding your personal cancer risk is key to empowering yourself to make informed health care decisions. The next few chapters will give you the tools you need to take control of your cancer risk.

Summary

To take control of your risk of cancer, it's helpful to know your personal risk. Several online calculators can provide you an estimate of your five-year or ten-year risk. It will help you put in perspective what you need to do to maximize your present and future health. Consider using one today and discuss the results with your doctor. Knowledge is power!

ANSWERS

1. **FALSE**—Although we can estimate your risk for some cancers, our predictions are not as accurate as we would like.

2. **TRUE**—Cancer-risk calculators have been primarily based on rates among whites. As a result, some of them may be less accurate in Blacks and Hispanics.

3. **TRUE**—Online calculators are for people at normal risk. People with known genetic mutations should not use the online calculators.

4. **TRUE**—As we get older, our risk for most cancers increases.

5. **FALSE**—Despite advances in cancer treatments, you should not assume you will be cured. Most therapies look at five-year survival rather than cures. Prevention is the best strategy.

CHAPTER THREE

How Important Are My Genes in Developing Cancer?

TRUE OR FALSE?

1. Genetics accounts for 50 percent of cancers.
2. Genetics tests can tell you whether you will get cancer.
3. Family history of cancer isn't as important anymore since cancer testing is so accurate.
4. If you're adopted, you shouldn't spend any time focusing on genetics.
5. Genetics testing is basically the same whether a doctor orders the test or you use an at-home testing kit.

(Answers at end of chapter)

"I DON'T NEED TO WORRY about cancer. I did one of those tests in the mail and it was negative." This was Jessica's response when I talked to her about cancer prevention. Jessica, a fifty-one -year-old mother of three, was not getting mammography on a regular basis and had missed several screening intervals. She wasn't concerned—because, in her mind, she was "protected" from cancer based on her genes. Several year later, in her mid-fifties, Jessica felt a lump in her armpit and ultimately was diagnosed with breast cancer. Luckily, she was responsive to chemotherapy and radiation, and she has recovered. Like many people, Jessica mistakenly believed that genetics played the biggest role in whether she would get cancer.

The reality is that for most people genetics plays a very small role in whether they get cancer. Jessica thought she was making a good decision by taking a genetic test, but Jessica experienced a disconnect, which many people do, in truly understanding what the tests currently can and cannot tell you.

"Should I get one of those genetic tests?" I get that question at least twice a month. Around the holidays it's almost every day, when the tests are often top sellers. Maybe you received one as a gift, and now you're wondering whether you should spit in a tube and send it in. When asked that question, I always reply with my own question—"Why do you want one?" Most times, I already know the answer. You want to know if you're going to get cancer.

One of the biggest and most harmful myths about cancer is that it's mostly genetic. The exact opposite is true. That's right—most cancer is not caused by our inherited genes. We are not predestined to get cancer. In fact, experts believe that only 15 to 20 percent of cancer cases are due to a direct effect of our inherited genetics. The rest is caused by your lifestyle choices—what you eat, how much you weigh, the quality of your sleep, amount of time in the sun, whether you smoke, and whether you exercise or not. Notice anything? These are all things that you have a lot of control over.

Fifteen to twenty percent is not zero, however. There are some types of cancer for which genetics does play a significant role. So, for some people, getting a genetic test might be a good idea. But the key is getting the right kind of test and truly understanding what the results mean.

Given the popularity of some of the direct-to-consumer tests, I'm going to break down the science and help you decide if these tests can play a role in your personal cancer prevention program.

Let's start with a quick genetic refresher that you probably haven't thought of since high school biology class. Genes are pieces of DNA inside our cells that tell our cells how to function. When cells divide and replicate, they sometimes make a mistake and then don't function properly. It's like a manufacturing assembly line—sometimes a product isn't made right. Mistakes happen for a variety of reasons. We have all purchased a product that turned out to be damaged when we opened the box. Genetics is the field of science that looks at how traits are passed down from parents to their children through genes. When you have a cancer that is "inherited," it means it resulted from a mutation (an error in copying the genetic code) that at least one of your parents or grandparents had. Usually, it had an "autosomal dominant" pattern of inheritance. I'm sure you have not heard that term in a long time! It means that you only need one parent to have the mutation, which gives you a 50 percent chance of inheriting the mutation. Having an inherited genetic mutation does not mean you will get cancer. It simply means you are at a higher risk for developing a certain type or types of cancer. The types of cancer that have a greater genetic connection usually result from a single genetic mutation. These include some types of colorectal, breast, ovarian, and pancreatic cancer.

The key point here is that if you are at increased risk, you need to know it, because you can still reduce your risk and your family's risk of developing cancer through screening and lifestyle changes. This is where genetic testing can play an important role.

If you're considering a genetic test, I suggest you compile a detailed family history of cancer before the test, not afterward. Your family history will help you (and your doctor) decide which test is best and how to interpret results. Compiling a detailed family history isn't easy. You do need to be a bit of a detective—but it is worth your time. In many

DEGREES OF FAMILY RELATIONSHIP

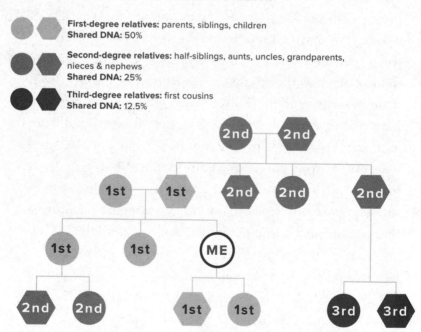

First-degree relatives: parents, siblings, children
Shared DNA: 50%

Second-degree relatives: half-siblings, aunts, uncles, grandparents, nieces & nephews
Shared DNA: 25%

Third-degree relatives: first cousins
Shared DNA: 12.5%

Figure 5

ways, a good family history is the best genetic test! Some key information is covered in Figure 5.

First-degree relatives in a genetic family history are those with no other family member between them. For example, child, parent, or sibling (they share 50 percent of their DNA).

Second-degree relatives in a genetic family history are those who have one family member between them. For example, grandparent and grandchild, half-siblings, aunt and uncle, and niece and nephew. (On average, they share 25 percent of their DNA.)

TAKING A GOOD and comprehensive family history doesn't have to be complicated. Here's what you should ask:

- Who had cancer and what type?
- Was that relative on your mother's or father's side?
- Are they a first-degree relative (mother, father, sister, brother, child)?
- How old were they when they were diagnosed?
- What is their race and ethnicity?
- Are they still living? If not, at what age did they die and what caused their death?
- Has anyone had genetic testing? (All too often, someone says, "Oh yea . . . they had it a couple years ago!") If so, find out those results.

Be sure to write the information down (either old-school with pen and paper or digitally) and include the date. Some apps out there can help with organizing this information. The CDC, American Medical Association, as well as the Office of the Surgeon General provide information on their sites to help create a family medical tree. Even though you are most interested in the health of first-degree relatives, go ahead and ask aunts, uncles, and cousins about their health, and what they know about your family members' health. Getting information on two or three generations can be especially useful when it comes to understanding your risk.

Make it a point to regather this information every couple of years. New information becomes available and sometimes family members become more aware later of information they might have forgotten. You might jog their memory. If nothing else, it will give you reason to reach out to your family members and catch up.

While you can't control what genes you have, you can control how much you know about your genetic background by obtaining a detailed family history. Remember: knowledge is power—so go get some power!

If you do find that some of your relatives had cancer, you might be thinking that cancer "runs in your family." I hear that a lot from patients, and from a genetic perspective, sometimes that's accurate, but sometimes it's not. For genetic causes, it does matter who, what, and when. There's a big difference in cancer risk from a first-degree relative versus second degree or third degree. Cancer can sometimes run in the family even if not caused by an inherited mutation. For example, shared environments or lifestyles—such as tobacco use, poor eating habits, lack of physical activity, exposure to occupational or geographical toxins—can cause similar cancers to develop among family members.

Let's deal with those cancer types that are genetically inherited. Should you be concerned if you have many relatives on one side of your family who have had the same type of cancer, or if family members have more than one type of cancer? It does raise a red flag. If some family members have had cancer at a younger age than normal for that type of cancer (often less than forty-five years of age) that's also concerning. If anyone in your family has had a rare case, that raises alarms too. By "rare," I mean conditions you don't often hear about because not many people get them. Retinoblastoma (cancer in the back of the eye), penile cancer, insulinomas (tumors in the pancreas), breast cancer in men, and some types of melanoma are examples. A more detailed list is at the end of this chapter.

Ethnicity is also an important consideration when looking at genetic risk since some mutations are more common in certain populations. For example, many women are aware that Ashkenazi (Eastern European) Jewish ancestry is linked to ovarian and breast cancers.

How Do You Pull All of This Together and Decide if You Should Get a Test?

Here are the four questions you need to ask as part of your personal cancer prevention program when considering genetic testing:

1. Should I get a test?
2. If so, which test?
3. What do the results mean?
4. If I do have risk, what is the likelihood that I will get cancer?

Should I Get a Test?

To answer that, first gather the family history that we just discussed. If you are at increased risk based on your family history, then you should seriously consider getting tested. If you're simply curious—as many people are—that's fine, too, if you know what the tests do and don't do, and how to interpret the results. Sometimes couples want genetic testing before conceiving, to know if they are at risk of passing along a variant to children. I completely understand those reasons, and being explicit up front about your reasons can help determine the type of test you take.

If you had trouble pulling together a thorough family history, ancestry tests might help you find people to whom you are related. By speaking with them (real or virtually), you may be able to gather more data about diseases that may run in your family. These tests can also help people who are adopted, who typically know very little about biological relatives. Identifying people to whom you are biologically related can help you, particularly if you've been adopted, to get a clear family history for many health conditions, including cancer.

If So, Which Test?

Different types of genetic tests have different purposes. The first looks for inherited or hereditary mutations that are passed down from your parents, grandparents, great-grandparents, and so on. The second—typically done after you have been diagnosed with cancer—looks at non-inherited mutations. Such mutations—EGFR (lung cancer) or CHEK2 (breast and colorectal cancer), for example—can occur randomly throughout your life. They may also be called biomarkers of cancer. This test can predict the effectiveness of certain treatments.

For purposes of your personal cancer prevention program, we are talking about the first type of test—the one looking for gene mutations in your family history. I know most people think of the over-the-counter tests such as 23andMe as well as AncestryDNA. These are known as direct-to-consumer tests (DTCs), meaning you don't need a doctor's prescription to get the test. You perform this test at home, typically by spitting into a tube, and the results come back directly to you in a couple of weeks. These at-home DTC tests are very limited in what they look for and, as with any test, it's important to know what they can and can't tell you.

There are now some DTC tests (Invitae, for example) that give you the option to speak to a physician when you request a test kit, and some will ask you some general health questions. A doctor—who is not your own—will review and authorize it. The results are still sent to you directly.

Another type of genetic testing is ordered by your doctor. These tests typically require a phlebotomist to draw your blood at a lab or in a clinic, and the results are sent directly to your doctor. These tests are much more comprehensive and accurate than the at-home tests, measuring for more potentially faulty genes that might cause cancer. An at-home test is not a substitute for in-office genetic testing. They are very different.

If you have compiled a strong family history, or if a family member took an at-home test and is concerned with the results—and you want to know about your own risk—you should consider skipping the at-home test and go directly to your doctor. Your doctor's tests provide more specific, better quality information. You may also want to consider speaking with a genetic professional either before you decide to take the test or about your results afterward. Genetic professionals are typically health care workers who have expertise in diseases that run in families. They provide counseling about genetic testing, and help to interpret the results.

Take time to think through what you really want to know as part of your personal cancer prevention program, and that will help guide your testing decision.

What Do the Results Mean?

The results of any genetic test can be difficult to understand. Trying to read them on your own can be harmful, since the information that's there might not tell the whole story, and you might misinterpret what you read. Even the words can be confusing and may have meanings that you won't understand. Positive, negative, true negative, uninformative negative, variant of uncertain insignificance, benign (harmless variant). Those aren't words you use every day, are they?

Whatever kind of genetic test you get, remember that these tests look for genetic risk—they do not diagnose cancer. A "positive" test doesn't mean you will automatically get cancer; and a "negative" test doesn't mean you won't ever get cancer. Negative tests are not a "get out of jail free" card that allows you to do whatever you want. Why? As I stated earlier, inherited cancers are a small percentage of the total number of new cancer cases—and deaths. Don't let a negative result give you a false sense of security.

When interpreting the results, keep in perspective which test you used. Why does that matter? There are a couple of important reasons. At-home genetic testing and in-office testing are not the same test and do not test for the same things. The at-home tests for cancer risk often involve the analysis of common inherited genetic variants that, individually, are generally associated with only a minor increase in risk. They do not test for every type of inherited form of cancer. In addition, some data suggests these tests are not as accurate in persons of non-European ancestry. Alternatively, doctors test for inherited genetic variants that are associated with a high to moderate increased risk of cancer.

It can seem like a lot of information, often in small print, but you must read the package insert that comes with the at-home test (or online at the product site). You want to know exactly what it tests for. I know many people think it tests for "cancer," but, to repeat, cancer is many different diseases, and these tests cover only a very limited number of them.

I was curious how the results are presented, so I compared two over-the-counter tests from two different companies. They can be confusing. Although no variants were detected, if I hadn't read the results carefully, I would have concluded that I'm unlikely to get cancer. The fine print does say that it doesn't include all possible variants with each condition, but I really had to pay attention.

So, what do tests like 23andMe cover? Most look for hereditary mutations that can cause breast cancer and a specific type of colon cancer syndrome. For breast cancer, it looks for three of more than one thousand known variants of BRCA1 and BRCA2, the two genes associated with hereditary breast cancer that often occurs earlier in life than some other types. They are also the three most common muta-tions in Jewish individuals. You read that correctly—some DTC tests currently look for only three of the most com-mon variant mutations of the BRCA genes, even though there are more than one thousand. That could lead to miss-ing a significant number of people who carried a BRCA mutation not detected by the test. In other words, a nega-tive test could still mean that you have an increased risk of cancer due to gene mutations. Detection of such cancer risk is vitally important.

BRCA MUTATION BREAST CANCER RISK	
POPULATION RISK	HEREDITARY RISK
0.6% for age 40	12–25% by age 40
2% for age 50	40–60% by age 50

Remember, mutations prevent genes from functioning properly. You likely have heard BRCA is related to breast cancer but it is also associated with ovarian cancer and some prostate cancer.

Keep in mind that no test is a comprehensive cancer strategy. They do not diagnose cancer and should not be used to make medical decisions about treatments. Please do not use them as a substitute for cancer screening. I have heard patients say, "I don't need a colonoscopy because my test said I'm not at risk for colon cancer." That is simply not what the test says and interpreting the result that way can lead to bad outcomes. A genetic test might reveal that you aren't at risk for hereditary colon cancer—not every type of colon cancer. It's important information, indeed, but you need to put it in the right perspective.

If I Do Have Risk, What Is the Likelihood That I Will Get Cancer?

If the test says you have a variant, no need to panic—having a variant doesn't mean that you will definitely develop cancer. Even when added together, all the known common variants associated with a particular cancer type account for only a small portion of a person's risk of that cancer. Remember this key point: most cases of cancer are not caused by hereditary gene mutations but by a wide variety of factors, including smoking, obesity, diet, and other lifestyle issues. The presence of a genetic mutation and variants are only one risk factor—albeit, for some cancers, an extremely relevant one.

How many family members have been affected by a variant? Your family history may indicate that variant's "strength." It makes a difference whether only one family member has cancer or multiple members do. And it matters if two or more cancers have occurred in the same relative. The scientific term is "penetrance." We also talk about how genes are "expressed." Think of it this way—people with the same faulty gene show different signs and experience different symptoms. We also know that lifestyle, as well as environmental risks, influence how genes—including faulty ones—work.

That's why it is so important to discuss your personal cancer risk with your doctor. I realize that, many times, you don't want to "bother" your doctor about it. Please do bother us! And don't bring it up at the end of a visit, but make your concern about cancer the whole point of the visit. That way, we can have a series of good discussions about next steps. You might even want to see a genetic counselor who has special training in evaluating your individual risk based on the test findings and your family history.

_____

Some Other Factors to Contemplate Before You Decide to Take a Test

The results of these tests—especially when positive—can affect other family members in different ways. You might be thinking you need to tell everyone, to "save them," especially since some family members may be likely to have the same mutation you do. But keep in mind that not everyone in your family, especially extended family, may be in the same mental or emotional place that you are. Some family members will want to know, and others won't. Family communication can have lots of complicated dynamics, can't they?! Ask whether they want to know before you share results.

You also need to be aware that tests can lead to more tests, and all this testing can then lead to stress and anxiety, as well as financial costs. Many of these tests can be several hundred dollars. Insurance might not cover everything, particularly if not ordered directly by a physician. Every type of test in medicine has pros and cons, so you want to weigh your decision carefully.

You also need to think about privacy issues—which can be complicated. It is illegal to discriminate based on genetic information, but, believe it or not, disability, long-term care, and life insurance are exempt from certain privacy laws and insurers are entitled to your test results. Whether it affects pricing of your insurance coverage is complicated, and always changing. Almost every year we see new federal and state legislation aimed at closing loopholes and making sure your genetic information is protected. Consider checking out the genetic information nondiscrimination act's website at ginahelp.org.

Summary

Genetic tests, including at-home tests without a prescription, can play an important role in your personal cancer prevention program. I know people want a "test for cancer," but the current at-home tests aren't the test that we really want, since they only tell a partial story as it relates to cancer. Some information, however, when interpreted correctly, is usually better than no information. It can provide useful information in certain circumstances to help you guide your decision-making and behavior as you strive to take control of your cancer risk. You do need to include these results in your health record, so everyone has the same information. Although today's tests are far from comprehensive, I do expect them to improve over the next few years. If you have a strong personal or family history of cancer, you should ask your doctor to order a test, since it will provide much more and better information.

In the meantime, if you are interested in trying an at-home genetic test, go ahead and spit in the tube. Just be sure to discuss the results with your doctor to get the most accurate interpretation of the data and guidance to apply the information in your cancer prevention strategy. That allows you to take the test and take control based on those personalized results!

MORE THAN FIFTY hereditary cancer syndromes have been described. You can find more about them at cancer.gov.

https://www.cancer.gov/about-cancer/causes-prevention/genetics/overview-pdq#_123

- Basal Cell Nevus Syndrome, Gorlin Syndrome, Gorlin-Goltz Syndrome, or Nevoid Basal Cell Carcinoma Syndrome
- Birt-Hogg-Dubé Syndrome
- Bloom Syndrome
- Breast/Gynecologic Cancers, Hereditary
- Brooke-Spiegler Syndrome
- Carney-Stratakis Syndrome
- Colon Cancer, Hereditary Nonpolyposis, or Lynch Syndrome
- Cowden Syndrome and PTEN Hamartoma Tumor Syndromes
- Dyskeratosis Congenita (Zinsser-Cole-Engman Syndrome)
- Epidermodysplasia Verruciformis
- Epidermolysis Bullosa
- Familial Cylindromatosis
- Fanconi Anemia
- Gastric Cancer, Diffuse and Lobular Breast Cancer
- Hyperparathyroidism, Familial
- Li-Fraumeni Syndrome
- Medullary Thyroid Cancer, Familial
- Melanoma, Hereditary

- Muir-Torre Syndrome
- Multiple Endocrine Neoplasia Type 1
- Multiple Endocrine Neoplasia Type 2A, 2B (Sipple Syndrome)
- Multiple Familial Trichoepithelioma
- Oculocutaneous Albinism
- Oligopolyposis
- Paraganglioma, Hereditary
- Peutz-Jeghers Syndrome
- Pheochromocytoma, Hereditary
- Polyposis, Familial Adenomatous, and Attenuated Familial Adenomatous Polyposis
- Polyposis, Familial Juvenile
- Polyposis, Hereditary Mixed
- Polyposis, MUTYH-Associated
- Polyposis, Serrated
- Prostate Cancer, Hereditary
- Renal Cell Cancer, Hereditary with Uterine Leiomyomas
- Renal Cell Cancer, Hereditary Papillary
- Rothmund-Thomson Syndrome
- Von Hippel-Lindau Syndrome
- Werner Syndrome
- Xeroderma Pigmentosum

ANSWERS

1. **FALSE**—Genetics likely accounts for less than 30 percent of cancer.

2. **FALSE**—Genetics tests do not tell you whether you will develop cancer, but typically tell you whether you have a specific mutation that may put you at risk for a type of cancer.

3. **FALSE**—Family history is one of the best genetic tests for cancer.

4. **FALSE**—Given widespread social media sites around ancestry and various genetic tests that allow you to share information, finding information about your genetic history, while harder when you are adopted, still provides you valuable information about your cancer risk.

5. **FALSE**—Genetics tests conducted through your doctor's office look for a greater number of mutations associated with certain cancers than at-home test kits, and provide more and better information.

CHAPTER 4

Which Screening Tests Do I Really Need?

TRUE OR FALSE?

1. Screening for cancer doesn't start until your forties.
2. You can't screen for most cancers.
3. When your doctor recommends cancer screening, it's because you might already have cancer.
4. If you are not a smoker, you don't need to be screened for lung cancer.
5. You can take a blood test to detect cancer.

(Answers at end of chapter)

"TIMING IS EVERYTHING." It's that combination of planning and chance that can have a significant impact on your life. Timing is key when it comes to job opportunities, relationships, home buying, and cancer prevention. Ideally, you want to catch cancer before it has grown much. To do that, you need to know what screening test you need, when you need it, and how often you should repeat it.

Patty is a fifty-two-year-old Asian friend of mine who often asks me medical questions—even though she has a primary care physician. Over the years, I have found that colleagues and friends sometimes feel more comfortable talking to me about their health issues than to their actual physician. Patty is in fairly good health, just taking some vitamins. She is always interested in discussing new technologies, especially those in the health field. "What do you think of the pill camera instead of a colonoscopy?" she asked one day. "I don't want a tube in my rectum." She was referring to a procedure in which a patient swallows a tiny camera—the size of a large lima bean—which transmits pictures of the intestine and then exits the body in a bowel movement. I responded based on her age and ethnicity. "Patty, you need a colonoscopy—either with the tube or the pill. You should have had one two years ago." I did add that I prefer colonoscopy since if you have a polyp, it can usually be removed the same day. Patty considered my advice but chose the pill camera. Unfortunately, the camera got stuck within her intestines. A CT scan followed by a surgery to retrieve and remove the capsule ultimately showed a small bowel sarcoma. Luckily it had not spread to other organs in her body. Patty underwent surgery, radiation, and immunotherapy and has been cancer-free for some time.

Patty always says she was "lucky" she chose the pill camera procedure, since it was the camera getting stuck that revealed her cancer. Maybe luck did play a role in a weird sort of way, but Patty did ultimately make the decision to be screened for cancer. I don't want people to be "lucky" to find cancer, but to follow the best screening recommendations we have, based on their personal cancer risk.

What Do We Mean by a "Screening Test" and What Do We Use Them For?

We use screening tests to find cancers—small and early-stage cancers, we hope—in people who have no symptoms. The reason why screening is so important is that it helps us find cancer before it spreads. By the time you have symptoms and you think something might be wrong, the cancer might have grown and spread, making treatment much more complicated. Timing is everything! It literally can make a difference between life and death.

Sounds like a pretty straightforward argument for screening, right? Still, many people don't get screened regularly, if at all. There are many reasons why, and you may be familiar with some of them. Maybe you feel you aren't at risk and the guidelines don't apply to you. Or you're concerned about the cost and/or the time needed to perform the screening. Perhaps you feel uncomfortable with tests such as mammograms and colonoscopies, or you feel embarrassed about taking your clothes off for a complete skin exam. Maybe you don't even know you are supposed to be screened. Or you got a screening test once and thought you were finished, and didn't need to have it done again.

It used to be that people would have an ongoing relationship with a primary care physician who would make these types of screening recommendations, but with the rise of the "doc in the box," those doctor-patient relationships are changing. Many people now only go to a doctor to treat symptoms when they develop, skipping checkups and missing out on preventive screenings for potential problems. Or they use "Dr. Google" to self-diagnose and treat. When you take this approach, you likely see a different doctor each time, so you don't develop the relationship that would lead a doctor to suggest screening. Your medical records might not be up-to-date, making it difficult to know what care you may need at what time.

These reasons are understandable, but screening tests are essential to your personalized cancer prevention program. By following the recommended screenings for cancer, based on your age and underlying risk factors (see Figure 6), you can greatly improve your chances of spotting cancer early, and may save your life. I'm going to help you learn which screening tests you need so you can take control of your cancer risk.

CANCER SCREENING FOR PERSONS AT AVERAGE RISK

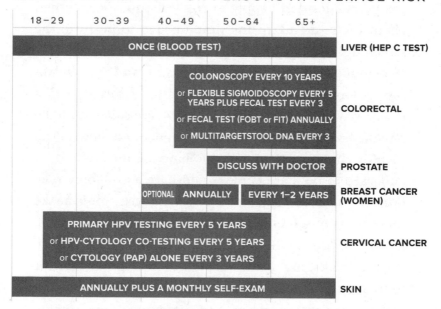

Figure 6

That said, it's important for you to know—up front—that, like any other tests, screening tests are imperfect and sometimes give the wrong results. For instance, you might get a false positive—that means the test says you may have cancer and you don't. If this happens, you might ultimately undergo several more tests until it's figured out you don't have cancer. That can result in psychological stress and added financial costs, and some of those additional tests could cause harm. The physical harm is usually minor—bleeding and soreness at a biopsy site, pain for a couple of days, or a scar that doesn't heal perfectly—but in rare circumstances it can be more serious: a heart attack or stroke, or even a perforation—a tear in a blood vessel or body part. That's a high price to pay for a test you don't need!

There also may be circumstances where finding the cancer doesn't change anything. By that I mean, treating it may not improve your health or make you live longer, especially if you weren't having any problems to begin with. Undergoing treatment might decrease your quality of life without lengthening it.

The screening test could also result in a false negative—that means the test says you don't have cancer, but you actually do. That's a big problem. You might delay seeking medical care, or assume you don't need any more screening, and the cancer might grow, making it harder to treat when it's finally discovered.

For the overwhelming majority of people, though, screening tests offer many more benefits than risks. We all know people who have had cancer, and even the less life-threatening varieties are no walk in the park. Some patients have remarked that they'll deal with cancer later if they get it. I don't think that's the right approach (and I bet their loved ones would agree). I'm going to take the right tests at the right time to prevent it, or to catch it early.

Unfortunately, a large percentage of people don't get the right tests at the right time. Less than 50 percent of Americans follow all the cancer screening recommendations. That's a low number, and it contributes to the death rate for cancer. If we want to decrease cancer deaths, people need to undergo the right screening.

Remember that when your doctor suggests a screening test, it does not mean he or she thinks you have cancer. Most of the time, the recommendations are based on age and/or family history. And screening tests are done when you have no cancer symptoms. Don't be like some patients I've had over the years who tell me they don't need screening since they don't have any symptoms. Or the ones that if a doctor recommends screening, they assume the worst and don't want to know. Remember, the best and most effective screening is done when you have no symptoms!

Do You Need to Be Screened?

Screening depends on several different factors that play a role in determining your risk. The most common include:

- Age
- Family history of cancer
- Gene mutations (such as BRCA)
- Exposure to cancer-causing agents such as tobacco or asbestos

People who have a high risk of cancer may need to be screened more often or at an earlier age than other people. More details on that in a little while.

Cancer screening tests shouldn't be treated like a cholesterol test, or a test for diabetes. This is not a "one size fits all" scenario. You want to have an informed discussion with your doctor about which screening tests are right for you based on your personal risk. If they don't take the time to discuss it with you, find a new doctor. Your doctor should make a recommendation about screening, but you should also be aware of what tests might be right for you.

Be sure to ask these questions:

- What's my personal risk for this cancer?
- When should I start screening?
- What are the benefits of screening, and do they vary by age?
- What harms from screening should I consider? Are they serious?
- How often do I need to be screened?
- When should I stop screening?

After you understand the benefits and harms of a screening test, you can decide whether you want to have the screening test based on what is best for you.

Let's look at current screening recommendations for some specific cancers.

Colorectal Cancer

The colon and rectum are essentially one big tube. The good news about colorectal cancer is that it is slow growing, so screening tests are very useful—but you must have them done! The bad news is that even though it's decreasing in people over sixty-five, colon cancer seems to be increasing among younger people. We are now seeing more cases in people in their thirties and forties, and even younger, which in the past was very unusual. We aren't sure why exactly that is; likely it's a combination of factors, including lack of exercise, poor diet, obesity, and other environmental components.

I know a lot of patients over the years who don't think about colon cancer screening because they tell me, "I don't have a family history." The statistics suggest this is a dangerous gamble. Only about 25 percent of colon cancers are related to genetics or family history. That means that roughly 75 percent—most colon cancer—occurs in people who have no family history.

In the past, the preparation for the screening was arguably worse than the test itself. The "prep"—the fluids and laxatives—that one had to take to literally "clear out the colon" were tough on the body. The good news is, we have made significant advances in colorectal screening. You have some screening options, but all are primarily looking for blood or a polyp/mass.

Colonoscopy. If there's one test that people don't show up for, it's usually a colonoscopy. "I forgot." "I didn't have anyone to drive me." "I had a headache." I've heard it all. I understand—the whole process feels a little yucky, doesn't it? You have to drink a bad-tasting solution, poop for several hours, and then have a tube inserted up your rectum. I had one done a few years ago. Like everyone else, I'm not looking forward to doing it again anytime soon. But I'm glad I did it. I had a couple of polyps removed, and it really solidified my determination to make sure I follow screening recommendations. To be honest, I didn't have it done exactly on time when I should have. I put if off as everyone else seems to be doing. As I look back on it, I'm so glad I finally had it done—especially since I needed to have a couple of polyps removed. These could have been malignant. The whole process was definitely worth it. And I'm happy to report the prep does keep getting a little easier. Depending on your results, you may not need another test for several more years.

I often talk about shared decision-making between physician and patient, which is when you decide together the best course of action. Colon cancer screening is a good example of the value of shared decision-making with your physician. After considering all the choices, I decided colonoscopy was the best choice for me, but it may not be for you. You do have choices. For instance, there is flexible sigmoidoscopy. It's like a colonoscopy, but it only goes to the left side of the colon where most colon cancers—but not all—form. You don't have to do as much prep, and you can usually stay awake—no anesthesia required. If the test is abnormal or you have polyps, you will then need a colonoscopy. So, if you go this route, be aware that you might end up having two procedures instead of one.

There's also the pill-camera procedure that Patty chose. You still have to do the same prep as you would for a colonoscopy, but there's no tube inserted, and you don't need anesthesia. You wear a recorder on your waist that captures the images from the camera. The camera comes out in your stool and is flushed down the toilet. Currently, the FDA has approved use of this device when the anatomy of a person's colon might make it difficult to use a colonoscope or there is an elevated risk of complications.

There are other screening tests that don't require a tube up through your rectum. But the screening interval time (when and how often to repeat) is different.

Fecal tests. These tests check for blood in your stool—often microscopic amounts you cannot see yourself. Colorectal cancer and polyps bleed, so the idea is that detecting blood would alert us to a problem. There are two types of fecal tests: the guaiac-based fecal occult blood test (gFOBT) and the fecal immunochemical test (FIT). The tests are similar. Both look for tiny amounts of blood in your poop, but the FIT tends to be more accurate and doesn't require changes to diet. It also looks for changes in DNA of your stool. One drawback, though, is that it does seem to cause more false positives than FOBT. With both tests, you take some samples of your stool from a bowel movement and send it into the lab. FOBT usually requires multiple samples. My issue with these tests is that colon cancer doesn't always bleed, so you can miss a cancer. And blood may be in your stool for reasons other than cancer, so a positive test doesn't mean you have cancer. Sometimes it's just hemorrhoids.

Stool DNA test. You might also hear this called multitargeted stool DNA test [MT-sDNA] or FIT-DNA. This is like the fecal test—you send stool samples to a lab—but in this test, the lab will also check for traces of cells from polyps or cancer by looking for changes in your genes. These have been advertised on television quite a bit in the last few years.

Double contrast barium enema. This is basically an X-ray of the colon and rectum. It still requires drinking a prep solution. It can give a good outline of the colon. Given some of the newer tests, this isn't as popular, and is rarely used anymore. The exception might be for people who cannot have a colonoscopy or other tests.

Patients often ask me about CT scans. Sometimes they are referred to as a "virtual colonoscopy." This test doesn't require a tube to be inserted into your rectum, and you don't need sedation. It combines X-rays and computer technology to create images of your colon. This technology has improved over the years in its ability to detect small tumors. Sometimes physicians will suggest this type of test when a patient cannot undergo colonoscopy. Part of the reason is that if there are any abnormalities noted, then a colonoscopy is still needed. That's why I'm a big fan of just getting the colonoscopy!

When Should You Start Getting Screened?

You should start getting screened at forty-five years old, but you might need to start earlier if you're at high risk for colorectal cancer. Note that this recommendation of forty-five years old was changed from fifty just a couple years ago, given the increased rate in younger people. The key is for both you and your physician to know if you are at average or high risk. Don't assume that your doctor will know this unless you tell her or him. Remember, family history is key!

The screening intervals for people at normal risk depend on the type of testing:

- Colonoscopy: once every ten years, or
- Flexible sigmoidoscopy every five years, plus a fecal test (FOBT or FIT) every three years, or
- Virtual colonoscopy every five years
- Fecal test (FOBT or FIT): every year, or
- Multitargetstool DNA (MT-sDNA, which combines a FIT test with a sDNA test) every three years

---

HIGH RISK CRITERIA FOR COLON CANCER

- A strong family history of colorectal cancer or certain types of polyps
- History of colorectal cancer or certain types of polyps
- History of inflammatory bowel disease (ulcerative colitis or Crohn's disease)
- Family history of a hereditary colorectal cancer syndrome such as familial adenomatous polyposis (FAP) or Lynch syndrome (also known as hereditary non-polyposis colon cancer or HNPCC)
- Radiation to the abdomen (belly) or pelvic area to treat another cancer

---

When Should You Stop Screening?

When to stop screening is a topic for discussion with your doctor. Given that it is a slow-growing cancer, if you have been up-to-date in getting your screening with no abnormal findings, we usually continue until about age seventy-five. There's no hard rule on this—much of it will depend on your underlying health.

Prostate Cancer

Prostate cancer is the second most common cancer in men. However, it doesn't typically occur in men younger than fifty. Over 60 percent of cases are diagnosed in men over sixty-five.

When I started my medical training, prostate specific antigen (PSA)—the lab test to screen for prostate cancer—was a routine lab that was ordered on all men over forty, every year! That's not the case anymore. We learned the PSA test is imprecise, often finding cancers that would not affect how long men would live, and the treatment side effects were considered by some to be worse than living with the cancer. For example, patients complained about incontinence, chronic pain, and impotence that sometimes occurred after treatment. Listening to the patients' experience made us rethink how we screen and treat. We needed to understand whether men were dying of prostate cancer or dying with prostate cancer. Over the last few years, we also learned more details about the pathology of prostate cancer, with some cases being very serious but others less so. Like other cancers, the stage at diagnosis plays a big role.

Again, screening is going to depend on your underlying risk—which is partly dependent on your age and family history.

Screening includes two tests:

Prostate specific antigen (PSA) test. As noted earlier, this is a blood test that tells us the level of a protein (PSA) released by prostate cells. Cancer causes the PSA level to rise, so if we see higher than normal numbers in the blood, it alerts us to the possibility of cancer. The problem is that other conditions, like an enlarged prostate or infection, can also raise those levels.

Digital rectal exam (DRE). If you're a male reading this chapter, you know what I'm referring to. During this test, you either bend forward while standing or lie on your side on an exam table. Then your doctor puts a lubricated, gloved finger into your rectum to feel for any lumps in your prostate. The doctor is trying to distinguish non-cancerous growth from cancer.

Both the PSA and the DRE are inexact, but right now they're all we have. They do give information, which can help with decision-making. A couple of new tests are under development, including one that analyzes urine, but these are still a few years away and need to undergo calibration and validation.

Different health groups have their own guidelines for prostate cancer screening. Your doctor can help you determine if you need screening, and if so, which tests you should have and how often to get them based on your underlying health. Please don't be tested without first discussing the risks and benefits of screening, as they apply to you.

I tend to support the advice of those groups that recommend most men get a PSA test, and possibly a DRE, around age fifty. Prostate cancer is more prevalent and more deadly in men of color, so if you're African American, or if you have a BRCA1 or BRCA2 mutation—or if there's a family history of prostate cancer in men younger than sixty-five—you may need to start testing as early as age forty-five. If you have more than one first-degree relative who has had cancer at an early age, then you could consider initiating screening at age forty. Depending on the PSA result, you might get retested every two years or every year.

Lung Cancer

It remains the deadliest cancer in men and women, even if it's not the most common anymore. Smoking is a big reason, so you should definitely get a screening test if you have a history of tobacco use. In fact, if you smoke, you are thirty times more likely to develop cancer and die than nonsmokers. Cigar and pipe smokers are also at increased risk. That being said, don't be misled into thinking smoking or secondhand smoke is the only cause of lung cancer, because it isn't. I have had many patients think they can't get lung cancer because they never smoked. But approximately 20 percent of people with lung cancer never smoked. Be aware that exposure to asbestos (surely you have seen the commercials relating to mesothelioma), radon, diesel fuel exhaust, as well as silica and coal products, increases risk of lung cancer. And if you had cancer and received radiation to your chest as part of your treatment, that can also increase your risk.

Chest X-rays are not a good screening tool for lung cancer. We used to do that a long time ago, but realized they often miss cancers, and if they do find them, the tumors are far along. CT scanning using low-dose radiation is now the preferred method to look for lung cancer, particularly in past and present smokers. It's a quick test that takes roughly a minute to complete.

In terms of who should be screened, recommendations have evolved over time as we've learned more. The most recent guidelines from the US Preventive Services Task Force, updated in 2020, recommended low-dose CT screening if you meet all of the following:

- Are fifty to eighty years old, and
- Have smoked at least a pack a day for twenty years (or an equal amount, such as two packs a day for ten years), and
- Smoke now, or you quit within the past fifteen years.

Just one in eight adults who meets these criteria receives screening, so it's important that you and your loved ones know about them. Given the impact of lung cancer on African American smokers, guidelines for screening can be more flexible, allowing for earlier screening. More than half of new lung cancer cases have already spread by the time they are diagnosed, so effective early screening is key.

Skin Cancer

Skin cancer is the most common cancer in the United States. More people are diagnosed with skin cancer each year—nearly three million people—than all other cancer combined. Approximately 20 percent of Americans develop skin cancer by the time they are seventy. Although it's common, when found early, patients with most types of skin cancer, especially melanoma, have a five-year survival rate of nearly 99 percent. When it has spread to surrounding areas, survival can drop to less than 20 percent. The key is preventing skin cancer and diagnosing it quickly. Skin cancer can be quite disfiguring, causing significant damage, so you don't want to ignore it, allowing it to grow.

When was the last time you had your entire body looked at for any suspicious moles or bumps? I bet many of you are saying "never." Several patients over the years have expressed surprise when I talk about the need for a complete skin exam. "Why do I need that?" has often been the response. The reason is it can be very difficult to see moles and rashes on areas such as your back and groin area.

Skin cancer can occur in some unexpected places. This includes inside the ear, under your fingernails, on your scalp or eyelids, as well as the soles of your feet. We need to be vigilant about these areas, but we often need someone else to help examine them.

Too often, people wait quite a while until a suspicious mole or "pimple" gets bigger. At that point, it's no longer screening. When I ask patients why they didn't come in sooner, they almost always say they didn't realize how big it was, or they couldn't see it that well, or they didn't think it was a big deal. "Doesn't everyone get moles when they get old?" is a common question, sadly often asked too late. The American Cancer Society says regular skin checks by your doctor are a good way to find skin cancers early, when they're easiest to treat. We need to examine its size, shape, color, and even texture—to help determine whether it's serious. We must closely look at sores that seem to bleed often or don't seem to heal. Your doctor should also feel for lymph nodes in your armpit and groin. If you've had the disease in the past, or you have family members who've had it, ask your doctor how often you should get a skin exam. Most people should have a yearly exam.

In between screenings, you should check your skin at least once a month. Suspicious spots that are cancerous don't go away, and usually change over time. That's why you need to check frequently. Use a mirror to look at those areas difficult to see—and don't forget the scalp! You might even need to ask a family member or friend to look on your back. Although most skin cancers occur in people older than sixty, some types of skin cancer can occur in people in their thirties. Don't think you are too young for skin cancer.

People of color develop skin cancers in areas that aren't commonly exposed to the sun more often than white people do. Many people of color also mistakenly believe they won't get skin cancer. As a result, they are often diagnosed at a later stage, which can make treatment more difficult.

I have seen too many patients over the years who waited too long to get a mole checked and were eventually diagnosed with advanced melanoma. That's what makes it so dangerous. Sometimes, it can be hard to figure out what is normal (especially "spots" we get as we age) versus what is cancerous. Many people don't realize that the cancer grows downward into your skin as well as above your skin. That's what makes it so deadly. When you have a question, check with an expert! I know people are also using some apps that allow you to take pictures and send them off to a dermatologist to review. These apps can be helpful in getting a quick assessment but don't rely exclusively on these results. If you find a suspicious spot, you still may need to go in to get checked since sometimes one needs to see the surrounding area as well as feel for those lymph nodes I mentioned earlier. If you are fair-skinned, have blue or green eyes, or naturally blond or red hair, you are at increased risk.

The other reason a skin exam is important is that some dermatologic conditions are associated with cancer. People with psoriasis have approximately a 20 percent increase in cancer—particularly skin, liver, pancreatic, and esophageal. The more severe the psoriasis, the greater the risk. Actinic keratoses—those dry, scaly rough patches of skin associated with too much sun—can sometimes turn into squamous cell cancer. There are good treatments for these conditions, but they still need to be examined by a dermatologist. Picking them off your skin is not a good idea and won't change any cancer risk that might exist.

What about those skin tags? We all get them, usually on our neck, eyelids, groin, or armpits. They are usually caused by friction and irritation with skin and clothing. Good news—these are not cancerous and, unless they are bothering you, do not require a doctor's visit.

Breast Cancer

Screening for breast cancer is an area where there is incredible passion and sometimes misinformation. One in eight women will develop breast cancer, so it is critically important to screen for breast cancer. It is the most commonly diagnosed cancer among Black women. Black women are also twice as likely as white women to be diagnosed with triple negative breast cancer, which means they lack estrogen receptors, progesterone receptors, and human epidermal growth factor receptors-2. This makes it more difficult to treat, so early detection is key.

Keep in mind that once you feel a lump, that's no longer considered "screening" because now we are trying to diagnose what it is, and you will undergo a different diagnostic regimen.

Most women are aware of mammograms, but confusion remains about the "right age" to start screening, as well as what's considered average risk.

When to Start

The American Cancer Society recommends women ages forty-five to fifty-four should have a yearly mammogram, although you could start as early as forty if you want to. Those fifty-five or older should get them every one to two years. Screening should continue while a woman is in good health and is expected to live ten more years or longer, although some data suggest annual screening if you are over seventy-five doesn't have a beneficial effect. Nearly half of women over age seventy continue to get mammograms, so be sure to talk to your doctor to see if you really need them.

These guidelines apply to women of average risk for breast cancer. I often hear people say the guidelines are wrong since "my mother died in her thirties." If that's the case, the guidelines don't apply, since you are not at average risk. If you're more likely to get breast cancer because of a family history or BRCA mutations, check with your doctor. You might need to have mammograms earlier and more often than these guidelines recommend. You may also need to add other screening tests, such as an MRI. MRI, however, does not replace mammography. Keep in mind that thermography—a technique that uses an infrared camera to look at blood flow—is not an alternative to mammograms either.

WOMEN AT HIGHER THAN AVERAGE RISK FOR BREAST CANCER

- Calculated lifetime risk of breast cancer of about 20 percent
- Documented BRCA1 or BRCA2 gene mutation
- A first-degree family member (including male) who's had breast cancer
- History of chest radiation
- Have Li-Fraumeni syndrome, Cowden syndrome, or Bannayan-Riley-Ruvalcaba syndrome, or have first-degree relatives with one of these syndromes
- Lobular carcinoma in situ (LCIS) or atypical hyperplasia

What about men and breast cancer? Breast cancer in men is rare. Male breast cancer represents less than 1 percent of breast cancer; fewer than 1 in 1,000 men will develop breast cancer in his lifetime. The mortality rate for breast cancer in men is higher than in women, however—likely because most men aren't aware of breast cancer in men and delay treatment if they do feel a lump. Most men don't think breast cancer is the cause even when they do feel a lump. Breast cancer screening is only recommended for some men at higher than average risk due to an inherited gene mutation (such as BRCA1 or BRCA2) or a strong family history of breast cancer. Men diagnosed with breast cancer are usually in their sixties.

If you're wondering about breast self-exams, most health groups don't recommend that women use self-exams as a preventive measure anymore. They cause many false alarms. If it's something you'd like to do to be familiar with your breasts, talk to your doctor about what you should look and feel for. It's important you do it correctly.

Cervical Cancer

This is one of the few cancers that starts pretty early in life—which can also be a barrier to detection because how many of us in our twenties are thinking that we need a cancer screening? We feel invincible! This cancer starts in cells that line the cervix, the lower part of your uterus. It is considered highly preventable through screening but needs to be caught early. Screening is critical since early-stage cervical cancer often has no symptoms. By the time vaginal bleeding or pelvic pain occurs during intercourse, cancer has often progressed to an advanced stage.

The American Cancer Society made some major changes in 2020 about screening. Instead of starting at age twenty-one, they now recommend age twenty-five. The preferred screening approach is primary HPV testing every five years through age sixty-five. If FDA-approved primary HPV testing is not available, then HPV-cytology co-testing every five years or cytology (PAP) alone every three years is acceptable.

These screening guidelines apply to all average-risk, asymptomatic people with a cervix, including transgender men who still have a cervix. Screening does not depend on sexual history or HPV vaccination status.

Women over age sixty-five who have had regular cervical cancer testing in the past ten years with normal results do not need to be tested for cervical cancer. Once testing is stopped, it should not be started again. Women with a history of a serious cervical pre-cancer should continue to be tested for at least twenty years after that diagnosis, even if testing goes past age sixty-five.

If you are a woman who has had her uterus and cervix removed (a total hysterectomy) for reasons not related to cervical cancer and who has no history of cervical cancer or serious pre-cancer, you should not be tested.

Some women—because of their health history (HIV infection, organ transplant, etc.)—may need a different screening schedule for cervical cancer.

Endometrial Cancer

Endometrial cancer occurs in the uterus—so screening depends on whether you still have a uterus. There are no screening tests for this type of cancer. That's why the American Cancer Society recommends that at the time of menopause, all women should be told about the risks and symptoms of endometrial cancer. The average age for endometrial cancer is around sixty years. Women should report any unexpected or unusual vaginal bleeding or spotting to her doctors. Pelvic pain or pain during intercourse can also be a symptom.

Some women—because of their history with Lynch syndrome, for example—may need to consider having a yearly endometrial biopsy as early as thirty years. Please talk with a health care provider about your history, to assess your risk.

Although white women are more likely to be diagnosed with endometrial cancer, Black women are much more likely to die from it.

Head and Neck Cancer

Don't forget that cancer can occur in these areas of the body. And they can be deadly! Screening for these cancers is typically done manually by your doctor. They should be feeling for lumps on your neck as well as looking in your mouth. I find many of my physician colleagues don't do this routinely, especially in the oral area. Dentists are very good at helping with this type of screening, and I have had quite a few referrals over the year from dentists for suspicious masses. Another reason to go see your dentist at least annually!

There are some trials looking at analysis of your breath to look for chemicals associated with tumors, but that's early on in development.

Tobacco and alcohol use are the major risk factors for head and neck cancers. Some other types of disease such as Fanconi anemia, HPV, Epstein-Barr virus, and Plummer-Vinson syndrome also increase your risk. If you experience gastroesophageal reflux disease, you should keep that under control since stomach acid going back in your throat might increase your odds of tumor growth.

Some data suggests that marijuana use might increase your odds of getting head and neck cancer, given the chemical composition of its smoke is similar to tobacco smoke, but more research needs to be done.

Liver Cancer

You may be thinking alcohol is the number one cause of liver cancer. You'd be wrong—the leading cause in the United States is hepatitis C.

Chronic hepatitis C causes inflammation, which then can lead to abnormal cell growth, which can then lead to cancer. The US Preventive Services Task Force now recommends screening for hepatitis C in all adults eighteen to seventy-nine without known liver disease. It's as simple as a blood test. Not only will it alert you to hepatitis C, but it acts as a preventive measure against liver cancer. And the great news is that hepatitis C is now curable.

Chronic hepatitis B can also cause inflammation, which might lead to liver cancer. Cirrhosis, often caused by alcohol abuse as well as a condition called hereditary hemochromatosis, also increases risk.

In terms of screening people at high risk for liver cancer, some doctors might measure alpha fetoprotein, which is often present in liver cancer but it's not very specific. Other doctors might recommend periodic ultrasounds.

•   •   •

I want to point out that not all cancers can be screened. For instance, pancreatic cancer has no screening plan. If someone has a strong family history or known genetic syndrome, then they might need a special ultrasound or MRI. Thyroid cancer is also not routinely screened. Your doctor should be palpating your neck during routine exams and might need to do ultrasounds based on findings. You might also be surprised we still don't have a good screening test for ovarian cancer. Remember, screening is a test used to look for disease when there aren't symptoms. If you have symptoms, it's no longer screening.

We have made remarkable advances in screening technologies during the last few years and will continue to do so. Numerous blood tests being studied might help identify early cancers before symptoms develop. Tumor cells rely on your blood to get nutrients to grow. By examining the blood for certain proteins or genetic material fragments, we might get a clue cancer is growing. Right now, it's still too early to use blood tests alone to screen for cancer. There's also research into whether detection of DNA and RNA of certain microbes in our gut can distinguish between people with cancer and those without. We do need to make sure that we don't "overdiagnose"—identify cancers that would never affect your life; you may suffer some complications and decreased quality of life by treating them.

Artificial intelligence (AI) is also helping to identify smaller tumors in the screening process and reduce the false positive rate as well as false negative rate. AI can look at X-rays and scans and "see" more suspicious patterns than a single radiologist can, and process much more information. AI will eventually allow screening to become much more personalized so we truly screen based on your unique risk.

Attention dog lovers! You might be interested in learning that there are numerous research studies going on using dogs to sniff out cancer. Dogs' sense of smell is quite powerful. Just as they are used to screen for drugs, they might be able to screen for tumor cells, especially if powered with AI. There's some preliminary, encouraging data but more work needs to be done.

For now, get informed first about your risk for certain cancers, review the current screening guidelines, and start a shared decision-making discussion with your physician.

Summary

For many people, just the thought of screening for cancer can remind us of our mortality. Most of us don't want to think about dying, but screening must be a key component of your personal cancer prevention program. Remember, it's something to do when you are healthy—at a time when you are probably not thinking about cancer. Because we lead busy lives, screening doesn't always get the priority it needs. But, if you do develop cancer, don't you want to catch it as early as possible, ideally when you are in good health? That's why you need to inform yourself (as you are doing by reading this book!) and discuss these screening recommendations with your doctor.

Remember, these are guidelines as opposed to strict rules. Let's also be realistic—we don't do everything we're supposed to do on time. So, if instead of every twelve months, you get your screening at fifteen or even sixteen months, you may still be safe. The problem is when it slips to two years or five years! If you are supposed to get a colonoscopy in your forties, and you don't do it until your fifties, that can be an issue. These longer time intervals can allow cancer to grow, and then you can have real problems. That's a "coulda woulda shoulda" that no one wants to live with.

ANSWERS

1. **FALSE**—Some people, based on their family history and genetic profile, will need to be screened for specific cancers much earlier than forty.

2. **TRUE**—We can only screen for a limited number of cancers. That's why lifestyle is so important.

3. **FALSE**—Screening is designed to catch cancer early on. When your doctor suggests screening, it does not mean he or she suspects cancer.

4. **TRUE**—Most, but not all, lung cancer is related to tobacco use. The recommended screening guidelines for lung cancer only apply to people who smoke or who have smoked.

5. **FALSE**—We do not have a blood test to detect cancer.

CHAPTER FIVE

Does Food Matter?

"I DON'T LIKE FISH. It smells fishy." That was my patient Bob's response when I suggested incorporating more fish in his diet. "The only fish I eat is fish sticks," he chuckled. I have been working with Bob for years trying to get him to eat more nutrient-dense food. "If you got rid of soda and instead drank water, you would probably lose ten pounds . . . easily," I recently told him. His response: "I don't like water. It has no taste." Bob has shot down every food suggestion I have given him. Bob is overweight, prediabetic, and hypertensive. He takes two medicines for blood pressure and one for high cholesterol. Bob hasn't made the connection yet between what he puts in his mouth and his overall health. It's a similar situation with Sylvia. She was recently diagnosed with diabetes. When I told her we likely could avoid insulin if we worked on what she ate, she told me, "Dr. Whyte, I've been fat for twenty years. And I've only been a diabetic for two months. I don't think what I'm eating is the problem."

When it comes to your health—including preventing cancer—I want you to realize that "Food is medicine." It's a phrase I've been using for decades—and even wrote a book about it. Food is truly as powerful and as important as pre-scription medicines. There's even on old proverb that says "he who takes his medicine and neglects his diet wastes the skills of his doctor." Food affects every organ and system in your body. Think about this—how do you feel after eating turkey on Thanksgiving Day? Or after eating a bunch of sugary sweets? I'm sure you know you don't feel the same after drinking a large cup of coffee versus multiple glasses of wine.

Food is the single most important factor for obesity. Sure, inactivity plays a big role too. Go ahead—run five miles a day and lift weights on the weekends. That will have multi-ple health benefits. But if you overeat by eating lots of food with low nutrients, you will still gain weight. Most people burn about 300 calories from thirty minutes on the ellipti-cal. That's admirable, but then when we consume a large order of fries with more than 400 calories, it becomes chal-lenging to keep the pounds off. It's an energy equation—how much energy we put in our body by the type and amounts of food versus the energy we put out in terms of types and intensity of different activities.

So, we need to think twice before we put something in our mouth. Should we have potato chips or a baked potato? An orange or a chocolate pretzel? When you consider food's impact over a lifetime, it really does matter. It's not about you eating chips today with your lunch, but rather you eating chips every other day for years. That's when the results of your choices become apparent. I have many patients who tell me they only eat ice cream occasionally—but when I push them for details, it becomes apparent that it's four days a week. I want you to think about the cumulative effect of unhealthy food choices—they catch up to us and cause problems.

Many people aren't aware of how powerfully food impacts their health because they've never been told. Nutrition hasn't been a subject that's been focused on in medical school, so many doctors aren't good at giving advice on healthy eating. They simply don't know the latest data. I've even had some patients ask me if nutrition really mattered, since none of their other doctors talk about it. "If food was so important, I would have heard about it," declared my patient Eileen when I urged her to cut back on her fast-food habit.

The reality is that food plays a major role in controlling your cancer risk. If your doctor is not educating you about nutrition, it becomes your responsibility to become informed.

The good news is we have learned over decades of research what foods might increase your risk of heart attacks, strokes, diabetes, as well as cancer. If you get diagnosed with diabetes—or even pre-diabetes—you start to change your diet. One of the first things that patients and their families do after a heart attack is "clean out" the kitchen of fatty foods. We do the same for numerous other health conditions such as gout and diverticulosis—we begin to realize how food can affect our health. Why can't we take the same approach for cancer? We haven't traditionally done that but we can start doing so today.

What we eat and what we die of are related. For instance, the incidence of colon cancer increases in Japanese men and women who move to the Unites States and change their diet from a fish- and plant-based diet to a meat- and carbohydrate-based diet. When it comes to your personal cancer prevention program, you want to do everything you can to reduce your risk, and that includes focusing on food. I want you to recognize that your risk of cancer and what you eat are related.

While a healthy diet can't completely prevent cancer, it can help reduce your odds of getting cancer. Just as you change your diet if you have diabetes or heart disease, you also need to change your diet to help prevent cancer. The same principles apply to many other health conditions. There are a few foods and concepts, however, that are particularly important when it comes to cancer. The foods you choose to eat create an environment in your body that can either promote cancer or prevent it. In a way, it's like what kind of fertilizer you are going to use: one to promote healthy cells or one that might cause unhealthy—cancerous—cells to grow. Which do you want to choose?

Let's start with foods that increase risk and you should likely limit. What do we know?

Red Meat

Red meat has consistently been shown to increase risk for cancer, particularly colon and rectal. Sometimes people ask me what exactly counts as "red meat." As its name implies, it is meat that appears red when it is uncooked. That means beef, of course, but also pork and lamb. Yes, contrary to what the marketers say, pork is considered red meat.

The connection to colon and rectal cancer seems to make sense because as meat is slowly digested, it comes into contact with the colon and rectum. It takes a while to chew and completely digest, so it is spending quite some time within our digestive system. That can increase your exposure to cancer-causing substances in the meat. But it's not just that part of your body that might be affected. There's also some data suggesting an increase in prostate and pancreatic cancer.

More research needs to be done as to why exactly red meat is associated with risk of cancer. It might be the fat content of the meat, or the cooking method. For example, when the meat is cooked at high temperatures or directly with a flame, harmful substances may be released that might cause inflammation and poison some of your cells, increasing the risk of a harmful mutation.

DOES CANCER RISK matter if beef is grass-fed or organic? In general, we believe that it is a healthier option to eat grass-fed meat since the animals graze freely on grass, which means they are not fed corn or soy. Organic means the animals are not given any hormones or antibiotics or exposed to pesticides.

That usually leads to a healthier fat content. Most grass-fed meat is organic. There's still a risk of cancer, but it is slightly lower with grass-fed meat; more studies need to be done.

Processed Meat

Processed meat is also another food that raises a red flag when it comes to cancer risk. Data suggests they increase your risk of colon, rectal, and stomach cancer—again those areas of our body involved with digestion. These foods include hot dogs, bologna, salami, sausages, and lunch meats. Is your mouth watering? The reason why these are so flavorful is they are salted, cured, or smoked for flavor and to help prolong shelf life. Sometimes the names of these processed meats in the supermarket makes them sound healthy, but they really aren't. Please don't be fooled.

The preservatives and chemicals used to process meat can change our cell metabolism, which then affects immunity. For instance, the nitrates that are used to keep processed meat fresher for longer could be converted into cancer-causing chemicals. Don't assume, though, that if you buy products that are "nitrates- or nitrites-free" that the risk is gone, because it is not. Nitrates or nitrites are not the only components that increase risk.

The association of cancer and meat consumption is fairly consistent, with numerous studies demonstrating the same findings of increased risk. The International Agency for Research on Cancer, an intergovernmental agency that conducts and coordinates research into the causes of cancer, puts processed meat in Group 1, which is carcinogenic, and red meat in Group 2A, which is "probably carcinogenic."

If you are at higher risk for some cancers, such as colon cancer, red meat, whether it's processed or not, might increase your risk even further. Knowing this can help you make the best decisions about whether you want to eat meat, what type, and how often.

Sugar-Sweetened Beverages

Soda, lemonade, fruit juice cocktails, sweet tea, and other sugary beverages may quench your thirst, but they won't help your health. Sugar-sweetened beverages don't directly increase your cancer risk, but their high-calorie content, which causes obesity, is likely to do so indirectly. They may also reduce our telomeres, which causes cells—including our immunity cells—to age and prematurely die, putting us at increased risk. Switching to the diet version may not eliminate the problem. Some data suggests that people who consume diet soda gain weight.

For instance, one study showed that participants who started out at a normal weight and drank three diet sodas a day were twice as likely as their non-diet-soda drinking peers to be overweight or obese eight years later. That seems counterintuitive, doesn't it?

There's a couple of reasons why we think this is the case. Those artificial sweeteners in the diet beverages are often much sweeter than sugar. That taste tricks your brain to tell your pancreas to release insulin. Then insulin makes you crave sugar. If you've been wondering why you crave a cupcake with that diet soda in the afternoon, that might be why!

There's also data to show that people overestimate their calorie savings from choosing diet beverages. How many of us have ordered a double cheeseburger and fries, and then said "diet coke" as if that somehow magically negates all those calories? I'm sorry to tell you it just doesn't work that way—I wish it did but, alas, it doesn't!

Here's a strategy that worked for me a couple years ago that might help you wean off diet beverages and replace any type of sweetened beverages with water. Try flavored water (adding lemon or lime) or sparkling water. There are plenty of fruit-infused waters on the market—there's likely one you will enjoy. Just make sure you choose one with no added sugar. Honestly, it will take some time to get used to the switch—possibly a week or two—but you can and should do it. Our desire for sugary drinks is learned—we aren't programmed at birth to want them. This also means we can unlearn these preferences!

Alcohol

Speaking of beverages, you may want to consider avoiding alcohol or at least cutting back. This includes wine. The impact of excessive alcohol on your health includes liver and brain damage, not to mention accidents—but it also affects your probability of getting cancer. An occasional drink is probably not too harmful, and doesn't likely affect cancer risk, but more than "occasionally" might have a different effect. Researchers in the UK estimate that drinking a bottle of wine a week (roughly one glass a day) is equivalent to smoking five to ten cigarettes in terms of impact on your risk for cancer. Alcohol consumption can account for about 6 percent of all cancers and 4 percent of all cancer deaths. Several studies have shown an increase in breast cancer in women who drink alcohol, even in small amounts. In their breast screening programs and clinics, doctors in the UK recognize this risk and counsel modifying a patient's alcohol consumption.

I bet you knew about the potential risk from red meat, but did you know about the association between alcohol and cancer? If you didn't, you're not alone. Awareness of alcohol as a risk factor for breast cancer is quite low. In addition, our ability to estimate how much alcohol we drink is poor; many people drink much more than they admit. Keep these estimates in mind because when it comes to breast cancer, alcohol increases risk, in a dose-dependent fashion—meaning the more alcohol you consume, the greater the risk. Data also shows that if you drink more than two or three alcoholic beverages daily, you may be 20 percent more likely to develop colon cancer.

I know a lot of readers might be thinking, "Hey, I thought red wine was good for my health." There was a belief several years ago that perhaps the resveratrol common in the grapes used for red wine could help protect your heart, and even improve blood pressure. Most follow-up studies haven't shown benefit, while the risks of too much wine—or any alcohol—are significant. And no group of guidelines suggests drinking red wine to improve your health. The studies on alcohol and cancer, particularly breast cancer, suggests it's the not the type of alcohol but the amount that puts someone at risk.

Highly Processed Foods and Refined Grains

This is probably not a surprise: prepackaged, processed foods are typically high in fat, salt, and sugar. This may help them taste better, but eating too many of these foods will lead to weight gain and might increase risks of some cancers. They often contain unhealthy additives such as hydrogenated oils, modified starches, colorants, and texturizers. You will improve your overall health if you eat fewer processed foods, especially those ultra-processed ones. As for refined grains, I'm not a fan. Refining takes out all the good stuff—fiber, vitamins, and minerals. Examples of refined grains include many breads, crackers, baked goods, and white rice. If you are like most people, processed and refined foods comprise a whopping 63 percent of the foods you eat. When you think about it, it's kind of insane that we take all the healthy ingredients out, and then add just a few back in. It should make you think twice about eating too much processed food and refined grains. They may not directly impact cancer risk, but shouldn't you choose foods to eat that have lots of nutrients rather than those that have had them removed?

I don't want you to read this and think you can never eat a hot dog or that by eating a steak and drinking a glass of wine, you're going to get cancer. That's not the case. Rather, your consistent choices over time determine your risk. If you eat steak and drink three glasses of wine every day, and drink soda all the time, you are likely increasing your risk of cancer as well as other chronic conditions. Food is medicine! What you put in your mouth is going to impact your body in ways that may take years to show. You likely won't feel the effects for some time. Remember Sylvia? She didn't realize that what she ate had a role in developing her diabetes. She ate whatever she wanted for a long time, but the effects of her diet choices caught up to her many years later.

What Should You Be Eating?

You can't just stop eating bad food and think that's enough. You also need to add good food.

What you include is as important as what you exclude. What should you be eating to help reduce cancer risk? There's no specific anti-cancer diet; rather, it's about types of food. The recently published guidelines from the American Cancer Society recommend including fruits and a variety of vegetables every day, favoring whole grains over refined grains, and consuming more fish instead of red meat.

That should be your goal. Remember, prevention is about making healthy choices most of the time. I know some experts say we need to eat a certain way, according to the guidelines, at every meal, but that doesn't work all the time for everyone. We don't want the perfect to be the enemy of the good. By this I mean, don't think you have to do everything right all the time to get the benefit. Don't adopt an "all or none" approach. That's just not realistic for most of us, and you will get quickly frustrated. Since most of us aren't eating as healthy as we should, even small changes gradually increased and improved over time can make a big difference in your personal cancer prevention program. The key is to start to focus on those foods that can help improve your body's immune response, decrease inflammation, and prevent tumors from forming or growing.

A simple way to do this is to shift more toward plant-based food rather than processed. Keep as close to nature as possible.

Let me break it down for you.

Fruits and Vegetables

If you're like most people, you probably need to eat more vegetables and fruits. They contain important vitamins and minerals, which may help fight cancer. I like them because they are high in fiber and low in calories—this helps you feel full with fewer calories, which can help you avoid overeating and becoming overweight. Of course, that assumes you aren't smothering the broccoli in melted cheese or dipping the strawberries in milk chocolate. ☺

As for vegetables, think variety including cruciferous ones! Some data suggests that cruciferous vegetables may help improve immunity. These include kale, arugula, collards, cauliflower, and bok choy. Chewing them raw, or lightly cooking, releases the chemicals our body might use to prevent cancer from growing. Broccoli and spinach should also be on your list as well as root vegetables such as beets and carrots. Several studies have shown a decreased rate in breast, lung, colorectal, and stomach cancer.

Fruits contain many important phytochemicals. We all know about vitamin C but that's only one benefit. For example, flavanones help to reduce inflammation. I sometimes hear from patients that they don't eat fruit because they are concerned about "sugar." The sugar in fruit is different from the sugar you add to your coffee or the one that is in candy and cakes. Most data supports the notion that the sugar in fruit does not cause a spike in blood sugar.

Honestly, I don't get too worried about someone eating too much fruit. It's always going to be a better choice than eating potato chips and candy bars. Fruit is Mother Nature's candy. In more than twenty years of practice, I haven't met one person who ate "too much" fruit. If you like candy, fruit is the way to go as part of your personal cancer prevention program. Be sure to go with the whole fruit, and not just fruit juices. Fruit juices have no fiber and are mostly sugar—the opposite of what you need.

Fish

When it comes to taking control of your cancer risk, one of the best dietary changes you can make is to replace some of those red meat meals, and eat fish instead—especially fatty fish such as salmon, tuna, trout, and halibut. Fish needs to be part of your personal cancer prevention program. It is full of omega-3 fatty acids as well as B vitamins and potassium, which may help to reduce inflammation in our bodies and protect cells. Like fruit, it's also low in calories, which is good for your waistline. Over the years, some folks have expressed concern about contaminants. For most people eating a variety of fish, either farmed or wild-caught, the levels of contaminants are too small to cause harm. Ahi tuna, tilefish, king mackerel, and swordfish tend to have higher mercury levels than other fish, so limit consumption of them. The benefits of eating fish, especially if eaten in moderation, are going to outweigh any risks. You should try to have at least two servings of fish per week—again, replacing red meat—not as a surf and turf!

You can also replace red meat with white meat a couple times a week, if you eat red meat regularly. Consider chicken, veal, and turkey. Several studies that examined this substitution demonstrated a decreased risk for cancer, including breast cancer.

Nuts

Do you ever eat nuts? I don't mean chocolate-covered almonds or the salted cashews. Nuts are a great source of protein and healthy fats. (Yes, some fats are healthy to eat!) Some, such as almonds and pistachios, even contain melatonin. You might be concerned that they have a lot of calories and they do, but moderation is key. Some research suggests that nuts, particularly walnuts, help to reduce inflammation and oxidative stress. They also contain some substances that help bind estrogen, which could reduce breast cancer. Go nuts over nuts! (Remember—peanuts are not nuts, they are legumes.)

Legumes

What is a legume? Sometimes I wonder if scientists make words difficult on purpose. Legumes mostly are plants that produce a pod with seeds inside. These include beans such as kidney and pinto, edamame, chickpeas, black-eyed peas, lima, fava, lentils, and soybeans. Legumes are more popular in some cultures than others and that might explain some ethnic differences in cancer rates. They are low in fat and have zero cholesterol but are rich in protein, fiber, iron, zinc, B vitamins, calcium, and potassium. Fiber, which most of us don't get enough of, helps our body repair DNA. It also helps feed bacteria in our gut that helps fight cancer cells. Another big benefit of legumes? Flavonoids, a type of plant compound, which research suggests might slow down tumor cells. Given this, consider making legumes a regular part of your diet. I think we are going to hear more about beans in the years ahead especially as we learn more about the role of our gut and the microbiome. The bacteria in our gut play a role in prevention of infections as well as our overall immunity. Some data suggests that people who are obese have different bacteria in their guts than people of normal weight have. Obese people may have fewer bacteria that reduce inflammation, creating an environment in which cancer cells can grow. We are just beginning to scratch the surface in this area of research.

Whole Grains

Whole grains are not something many of us grew up with. We were used to eating sandwiches on white bread for lunch. Some of us are still used to that, but it might be time to try something new.

What are whole grains and why do they matter? Whole grains include all or parts of the original kernel. It's "whole" because it is not refined or processed. That's important because it has much more fiber and vitamins than processed or refined grains. (Remember, the process of refining removes all the good stuff!) Whole grains also contain phenols that may help protect against colon cancer, as well as liver cancer. Part of the benefit might be related to the fiber in whole grains—which most of us don't get enough of— that helps keep us regular in our bowel movements. One study, which followed more than 125,000 adults for around 24 years, showed that the risk of liver cancer was 37 percent lower among those who consumed the most whole grains.

When shopping, don't be misled by labels that say "multi-grain" or "12 grain." Look specifically for "whole" to get the most benefit.

Seeds

When is the last time you ate seeds? Like nuts, they can be a healthy snack, and a much better choice than eating cookies. I remember eating sunflower seeds when I was young—but that was a while ago. Seeds, such as pumpkin, sesame, and chia, provide the vitamins and minerals that can help our DNA repair itself if it becomes damaged, an important strategy in cancer prevention. Seeds can have a lot of added salt, so go with unsalted or lightly salted. I'm a fan of flaxseeds in a shake, since it might help reduce your cholesterol and your risk of cancer. Go with ground rather than whole; it's easier to digest and you will absorb more of the benefits.

Herbs and Spices

Experimenting with flavoring is one of the most fun parts of cooking. Spices and herbs allow us to color foods and make it more flavorful. They might also help reduce your risk of cancer. They have been part of culinary traditions for thousands of years, and many cultures have also used them for their medicinal qualities.

I bet many of you have tried ginger ale when you had an upset stomach. Although many current soda products do not have real ginger, this spice had been used to help prevent nausea in patients undergoing chemotherapy before we had new drugs. Ginger also exhibits properties that prevent tumor cells from growing. Other spices such as saffron, turmeric, rosemary, and cumin may also stop cancer from growing by preventing blood vessels that feed cancer cells from forming.

Culinary herbs and spices may change some of the ways our cells work and how tumors behave. For instance, they decrease those bad free radicals and inhibit the ability of cancer cells to reproduce. They can help get rid of harmful bacteria and even strengthen our immunity to defend against tumors. Ounce for ounce, they have some of the highest antioxidant levels of any food group.

I bet you have overlooked garlic as part of your cancer prevention program. Garlic and onions can block the formation of nitrosamines, which have been implicated in colon, liver, and breast cancer. Some studies show that garlic can inhibit H. pylori activity in your stomach. These bacteria often cause ulcer disease, but can also be associated with stomach cancer. To get the most benefit, peel and chop the cloves and let them sit fifteen to twenty minutes before cooking. This activates enzymes and releases the sulfur-containing compounds that have protective effects, such as preventing cancer cells from replicating as well as causing them to die. Go ahead and stink up the kitchen! The World Health Organization recommends adults consume one clove of garlic daily to promote health.

More than 150 spices and herbs are available in most grocery stores. Have fun and do some experimenting! Why use processed and refined foods when you can create your meals with your own flavors? Believe me—you will notice a difference.

Dairy

The role of dairy in cancer prevention is contentious, and people on both sides of the debate are passionate. Some studies have shown an increase in breast and prostate cancer in people who consume high quantities of dairy while others have shown a decrease in colon cancer. One hypothesis suggests that milk from lactating, pregnant cows might be the cause for cancers such as prostate and breast that are hormone-dependent. The most recent data shows that most people benefit from dairy. Dairy does have lots of calcium and vitamin D—both of which seem to help with immunity. Remember, vitamin D helps with calcium absorption. Because of the high fat content of some products, I do recommend that you choose low-fat dairy, and keep to less than two servings a day.

Superfoods

I know "superfoods" isn't a real medical term, but the concept is a good one. When making food choices as part of your personal cancer prevention program, some foods are better choices than others and some foods seem to have special properties that might be protective. When you are deciding what to eat, you might want to consider some of these foods . . . which I do think are super!

Blueberries are one of my favorite superfoods. I try to eat them every day, often in plain Greek yogurt or oatmeal. They've got antioxidants, potassium, polyphenols, and vitamin C. This helps your cells defend against attacks from tumors, so they're at the top of my list.

For all you coffee drinkers, there's good news! When you look at the totality of the evidence, it demonstrates regular coffee—not the Frappuccinos and mocha lattes!—improves your health and cuts the risk of cancer when limited to less than two cups a day. The coffee bean does have antioxidants, which helps protect our cells from damage. It may also prevent new blood vessels from forming that cancer cells need to nourish themselves. It also speeds up our digestion, decreasing the time food is exposed to our stomach and intestines. Some preliminary data points to a reduction in cancer risk, especially for colorectal and liver cancer. It may also help people who already have cancer. Like everything else, coffee can be super if used in moderation—and not loaded up with sugars! All that sugar will just add on the pounds and defeat the health benefits.

THOSE OF YOU who live in California may remember that, in March 2018, a California court ruled that coffee companies in California needed to warn consumers that a chemical formed during the roasting process, acrylamide, was potentially carcinogenic. But since then the state's environmental health arm has argued that the latest research does not show that acrylamide in coffee poses a significant cancer risk.

For those of you that don't like coffee or want to try something different, I've got a good option—tea! More than two-thirds of the world's population drink tea. The leaves of the tea plant are rich in the polyphenol catechin, which keeps free radicals from damaging cells. Some preliminary data shows catechins can shrink tumors and reduce tumor cell growth, probably by suppressing certain harmful enzymes. The polyphenol's antifungal and antibacterial properties also fight infection, including in our digestive tracts.

Most of the health benefits have been studied in green and black tea, especially in reducing liver, breast, skin, lung, and pancreatic cancer. Be sure to let tea brew for about ten minutes to extract all those cancer-fighting molecules! If you're concerned about caffeine, note that green tea has less caffeine than black tea, which has less caffeine than coffee.

Ginseng tea may also be helpful in reducing the risk of certain cancers. Ginsenosides in this herb may help your immune system by reducing inflammation, lowering cortisol, and preventing growth of tumor cells. Some people have had allergic reactions to ginseng, so I do not recommend you drink it daily over long periods of time. Another tip is to drink it before a meal, which might help with absorption of those protective chemicals.

Consider this quote from William Gladstone if you are on the fence about trying tea: "If you are cold, tea will warm you. If you are too heated, it will cool you. If you are depressed, it will cheer you. If you are excited, it will calm you."

Another superfood I'd like you to consider is tomatoes. We have known for a long time that tomatoes contain the antioxidant lycopene as well as vitamins such as A, C, and E. It's the lycopene that gives tomatoes their color. There are several good studies that suggest lycopene might reduce the risk of prostate cancer. As someone with Italian heritage, I've always enjoyed tomatoes. And if you are trying to incorporate tomatoes in your diet, salads are a great idea, but tomato sauce counts too! Just watch the sugar content of sauces. Here's a tip when it comes to tomatoes and health: cook them to release more lycopene. Use some olive oil and get double benefit. If you don't like tomatoes, watermelon, papaya, and pink grapefruit also have lycopene. And for all you trivia fans: tomatoes are considered a fruit and a vegetable!

Grapes are another one of my favorite superfoods. Grapes contain activin, which may prevent cancer cells from invading your organs. They may even reduce DNA damage and prevent overproduction of free radicals. When there are too many free radicals, they start to damage normal cells. We used to think the color of the grapes mattered. Red, black, or green? Any one of them can be part of your cancer prevention diet. Fun bonus: they might even improve the quality of your skin!

When it comes to apples, an apple a day keeps the doctor away . . . but does it keep cancer away? Apples have an abundance of phytochemicals, which seem to have anti-cancer properties. Some studies in Italy—where apparently apples are very popular—suggest decreased rates in several cancers. We still need more research, but apples are always a healthy treat.

How Much Exactly of "Healthy Food" Do You Need?

The key is to make healthy choices over time, and incorporate some of them every day, as best as you can. Don't get bogged down in numbers, but look at the total picture of what you consume most days of the week.

Many people aren't sure how much fruit and vegetables they need to be eating. I can tell you the formal recommendations of two to three cups of vegetables and one to two cups of fruit daily. But most of us, including me, aren't that good at measurements. Is a big banana considered one cup or two? What if it's a large one or small one? Honestly, I think we make healthy eating overly complicated. Instead of worrying about measurements, simply focus on eating fruits and vegetables with at least two meals of the day. Many people don't eat any fruits and vegetables at all some days. Even if you start with one meal a day, you're making progress. More fruit is better when it comes to preventing cancer, but some is better than none. By the way, it doesn't matter much whether fresh, frozen, or canned. They're all going to be a better choice than processed foods.

In recent years, I've been asked about intermittent fasting. Some people believe that we need to "starve" cancer cells—especially of sugar. There's some data to support intermittent fasting for weight loss—a good thing, if you're overweight, since decreasing excess pounds will decrease cancer risk. But intermittent fasting will not kill cancer cells. If you decide to try fasting, just make sure you are still eating healthy food, and not just consuming fewer calories of junk food. Some techniques simply restrict the time one can eat and don't address the quality of food consumed. Remember, food quality matters!

What about the keto diet for cancer prevention? In some ways, it's the same idea: starve cancer cells of nutrients while providing fatty acids to sustain normal cell growth. But no data supports this hypothesis and no medical or cancer group specifically recommends the keto diet to prevent or treat cancer. Periodically the "alkaline diet" has been similarly popular as a cancer prevention strategy. The diet purports to create an alkaline environment that is harmful to tumors—but food does not control whether your body or blood is acidic or alkaline.

Be wary of fads. Instead, find a healthy way to eat nearly every day of your life. (Exceptions are allowed every now and then!) Choose foods that are going to create a hostile environment for cancer cells rather than those that help them grow. Remember, food is medicine!

Labels

I'm not a fan of counting calories. It works for many people, but for others it's not the way we think about eating. Rather, I'm big on comparing labels. So, if you are choosing between two yogurts (and you should be trying to eat yogurt some days!), you can simply compare both labels. If one has 22 gm of sugar and the other has 10 gm, you should choose the one with less sugar. You know the right choice if one product has 14 gm of protein and another has 6 gm. (Hint: pick the one with more protein!) If one brand has ten words in the ingredients you can't pronounce, choose another whose ingredients you know. Try it the next time you go grocery shopping! Your shopping cart might look very different.

Supplements

Should you consider the use of supplements in your cancer prevention program? Although sometimes supplements seem to be marketed as drugs, they are regulated as a food. That means they don't have to undergo any studies to prove safety and efficacy before they can appear in the store. That's important to keep in mind when you see ads proclaiming "prostate health" or "improved memory." If you look closely, there's always this tiny fine print that says such claims have not been evaluated by the US Food and Drug Administration. That's something you should think about.

Nearly half of all Americans take some type of supplement daily. But do you need them to help prevent cancer? I guess in theory it sounds good if you can increase vitamins and micronutrients—even artificially through a pill, it would be helpful. But I always tell people that if you eat healthy, you don't need to spend money on supplements. Also keep in mind that vitamins and minerals such as calcium, vitamin D, or vitamin C in a pill form aren't treated the same way by the body. In addition, more is not always better, and I have seen instances over the years where people develop health issues by taking a megadose of certain supplements.

Many of my patients don't tell me if they are taking supplements. "I didn't think it was important to mention. They're just over the counter," is often the reply. Don't assume that because you can buy it directly or it is labeled "natural" that it is safe. We have an attitude that "it can't hurt" but the reality is that everything we put in our mouth can have potential harm and benefits. Some supplements might also interfere with prescription medicines you are taking. It's always a good idea to tell your doctor what supplements, if any, you are using.

For those of you that don't like fish, you may be wondering about omega-3 supplements. First, I'd say there are lots of different fish to try and I encourage you to make an effort. Sometimes people will say that they don't like fish, but they really haven't tried it. You really must try a new flavor or food at least seven times to see if you like it. Or there's a fear of cooking fish. People think it's complicated when it's really quite simple and fast. For those that just can't do fish, an omega-3 supplement may be of value. It doesn't have all the same health benefits of eating fish, but it can help you get important cancer prevention benefits of fish oil. Just remember, that doesn't mean you can still eat all the red meat you want if you add fish or omega-3 supplements.

With supplements, there's also a danger of "too much of a seemingly good thing." Recent studies have shown that too much beta carotene, or vitamins A and E, increase risks of some cancers. For example, a couple of trials showed that people at risk for lung cancer increase their risk if they take high-dose beta carotene supplements. We used to think vitamin E and selenium could help prevent cancer, but the Selenium and Vitamin E Cancer Prevention Trial suggested they increased risk of prostate cancer. We aren't sure why. Some data shows that supplements may reduce the effectiveness of chemotherapy. So please don't think that taking lots of supplements doesn't cause any harm—because it might. I don't recommend taking supplements unless there's a good reason to do so, and your doctor recommends it.

During the last few years I've noticed a lot of interest in vitamin D and its potential impact on immunity. Trials have not shown that it's effective for cancer prevention. A very large trial called the Women's Health Initiative looked at whether calcium supplements and vitamin D affected colorectal cancer—they didn't. Yet, many companies still promote vitamin D supplements as boosting immunity. It may be helpful for bone health but it probably won't change your odds of getting cancer. My approach is always, "Let's do the trial and see if it works."

That's exactly what they did for the potential role of vitamin A intake and cutaneous squamous cell cancer, a type of skin cancer. In this cohort study of 48,400 US men and 75,170 US women, during a follow-up period of more than twenty-six years, higher total vitamin A intake was associated with a reduction in cutaneous squamous cell carcinoma risk.

You might remember ginkgo biloba being promoted as protecting against memory loss and dementia. Well, numerous studies showed it doesn't protect your brain. I always suggest that patients research supplements before they start taking any. Make sure that you are represented in populations being studied (a study may be limited by age, gender, or ethnicity, for example). I don't want you to waste your money, or, worse, put your health at risk.

What about probiotics? Or prebiotics? And what's their potential role in cancer prevention? They are plant fibers that help good microorganisms grow in your gut. They are "pre" since they are "before" the organisms are formed. Probiotics are the live bacteria and yeast we consume to help keep healthy bacteria and other organisms in our gut. You often see them in some yogurt and kimchi. By consuming more prebiotics and probiotics, you might outnumber the bad bacteria that cause infections. As it relates to cancer, they help reduce harmful cellular swelling and turn on cells called phagocytes, which eat and destroy bad cells. Nevertheless, we need more data before we can recommend these as part of a cancer prevention program.

Probiotics have other uses, but talk to your doctor before you start taking them. Some people can develop allergic reactions to probiotics, so be sure to consume small amounts at first.

Finally, don't have a philosophy that you can eat poorly and then fix that with supplements. No supplement will balance out a bad diet. Instead, focus on how you can make changes to your diet to include foods that are packed with nutrients. Such an approach will allow you to take control of your cancer risk.

What About a Food Journal?

Keeping a food journal is simple although somewhat tedious: you write down everything you put in your mouth. Sometimes I recommend that patients keep a food journal, at least for a week, to give them a clear view of what, and how much, they are eating—often very different from what they remember. I like to review the journal at the end of the week to see where one can make healthy changes. When you write everything down, and see that you only had two pieces of fruit and three vegetables over an entire week, it's easy to see how you can improve. Feedback is important when you are trying to make changes to what you eat. There are even different sites that will give you a nutritional assessment of what you ate (such as the National Cancer Institute's Automated Self-Administered 24-Hour Dietary Assessment tool). For those of you that are tech savvy, there are a host of digital trackers and apps that can help you keep an accounting with a food log, including estimated total calories. It's worth the time and effort to do at some point, to get the important feedback that can help you make additional changes.

Flush Bad Food Out?

I have known patients—and friends—over the years who believe that they can eat what they want and then occasionally "purge their body" with enemas and "detox" diets. Our bodies just don't work that way. Our liver and our kidneys serve the main role of getting rid of toxins. Such diets and cleanses can be dangerous, leading to dehydration, skin breakdown, and loss of important electrolytes. Instead of trying to flush bad foods out of your system, try not to put them into it in the first place.

> SHOULD I WORRY about the pesticides used in farming? Numerous studies have shown that the trace amounts of pesticides on fruits and vegetables do not cause harm. It's not a bad idea to rinse them before eating. The benefits of consuming fruits and vegetables far exceed any risk.

Summary

When it comes to food and cancer prevention, it's important to remember the following:

1. Food is as powerful as a prescription drug.
2. What you include matters as much as what you exclude.

Your dietary goals for your personal cancer prevention program are to eliminate foods that may promote mutations that cause tumor cell growth and include foods that boost immunity. Cut back on red meat, processed and refined grains, alcohol, and sugary (and so-called diet) beverages. Instead, to help reduce cancer risk, add healthy foods such as fruits and vegetables, whole grains, and fish to your daily meals. Pay attention to how you cook food and use spices and herbs liberally! Think about whether you are putting "high quality" food in your mouth every time you eat. You don't need to be perfect every day, but "exceptions" shouldn't become the rule. Think "big picture." Food's impact on cancer risk is generally slow and cumulative, over many years—so you have time to change your risk by changing what you eat.

I do think that in a few years science will evolve so that we will have "precision nutrition." That will tell us which foods we should eat based on our genetics and lifestyle. We aren't there yet, so let's do the best we can in choosing foods that help fight cancer.

WHAT ABOUT THOSE PLANT-BASED BURGERS? DO THEY AFFECT YOUR CANCER RISK?

These burgers are not meat but designed to look and feel like a regular meat burger. Since they are mostly plant-based, it seems like that should be healthy, right? Well, it's not quite that simple. "Elevation," "Beyond Meat," "Impossible," and other popular burgers mimic meat but they're not truly "veggie burgers," which are made of veggies and other natural ingredients, low in calories, low in fat and sodium, and high in antioxidants.

Rather, these burgers typically include plant protein but also peas, salt, food starch, and beet juice extract or modified heme to make it look like the color of a typical burger. You may be surprised to hear that they aren't much healthier than beef burgers. They often have the same amount of saturated fat and sodium and around the same number of calories. It's the calories and fat that I get concerned about, especially as they relate to obesity. Bottom line: probably a slightly better choice, but don't count it as one of your healthy meals!

DOES SOY CAUSE CANCER?

Soy-based foods have been popular at different times. Perhaps you are using soy milk in your coffee or incorporating tofu, edamame, or tempeh in your daily meals? Soy does contain phytoestrogens, plant chemicals that are similar to estrogen. This has caused concerns that people with hormone-dependent cancers, such as breast cancer, could be at risk. The most recent studies have shown that soy food does not increase cancer risk. Some soy foods do raise estrogen levels in the body, while others block estrogen. This research did not assess supplements. The key is moderation. Note this does not apply to soy sauce— which has little actual soy but lots of salt!

ANSWERS

1. **FALSE**—Red meat has consistently been shown to increase risk of colon cancer, but we need more data about other cancers. It's still a good idea to decrease daily consumption of red meat.

2. **FALSE**—No data supports the claim that vitamin D supplements protect against cancer. Eat a healthy diet. Talk to your doctor about getting a vitamin D level test and whether you need supplementation for a specific health reason, other than cancer. Don't just start taking vitamin D supplements as part of a cancer prevention strategy.

3. **FALSE**—Even small amounts of alcohol can increase risk of some cancers, particularly breast cancer.

4. **TRUE**—Although no one food prevents cancer, we do know that garlic contains numerous cancer-preventing compounds; incorporating garlic into your diet plan can decrease your cancer risk.

5. **FALSE**—Diet beverages often result in weight gain.

CHAPTER SIX

What Type of Exercise Makes Cancer Less Likely?

TRUE OR FALSE?

1. Lack of exercise increases your cancer risk.
2. You only need to do "cardio" to get benefit from exercise.
3. Exercise only helps prevent cancer if you are overweight.
4. Too much exercise can be harmful to your immune system.
5. Just twenty minutes of daily exercise is enough to benefit your health.

(Answers at end of chapter)

"I need to get in shape before I can go to the gym."

—ROBERT R, *fifty-five-year-old office worker*

"I just paid a lot of money to get my hair done. I can't be sweating."

—SYLVIA L, *thirty-two-year-old pharmacist*

"I walk around the office all day. Doesn't that count?"

—JIM Z, *sixty-year-old accountant*

"I can't afford a trainer."

—TERESA M, *twenty-four-year-old fast food-worker*

"I have no time to exercise."

—VANESSA G, *fifty-year-old web designer and mother of three*

"I don't feel like getting changed."

—JENNIFER R, *forty-two-year-old marketing executive*

IF YOU'RE NOT EXERCISING, you are not alone. Less than 5 percent of adults devote thirty minutes to physical activity each day, and only one in three adults performs the recommended amount of physical activity each week. It doesn't get easier as we get older. Only 28 to 34 percent of adults ages sixty-five to seventy-four are physically active. More than 80 percent of us do not meet the suggested minimums for aerobic and muscle-strengthening activities. What most of us don't understand is that when we avoid exercise (perhaps using some of the excuses I listed above), we're missing out on life-changing benefits as well as a potential decrease in the odds of getting cancer.

Exercise might be as close to a "magic pill" for a longer, healthier, cancer-free life as we'll ever get. Exercise has a powerful effect, not just on our bodies but also our minds. It improves muscle strength and endurance, while preventing muscle wasting. It builds bone density and lowers your blood pressure. It increases energy levels, and even releases endorphins—those "feel good" hormones that make you happy and reduce anxiety and depression. As long as you don't do it before bedtime, it improves your sleep. It also plays a big role in our metabolism, affecting our blood sugar level and rate of digestion. Exercise can determine the shape of our body, how much we weigh, and how much fat we have. Exercise also improves immune function and reduces inflammation, which is at the root of many modern-day diseases. It's during exercise that our lymph circulation gets rid of toxins. Research shows it can improve our thinking and our memory. It truly can make us stronger physically and mentally. Yet, we often find excuses not to exercise.

It is an important component in disease prevention and treatment. Our treatment of heart disease may be the best-known example. We all know that exercise protects our heart, don't we? Even the language we use to describe some exercises implies benefits to the heart. We say we are going to "do cardio"—its very name signifies we are protecting our heart! Cardiac rehabilitation, focusing on returning people to physical activity after a heart attack, so they can regain heart health and prevent future heart attacks, is a thriving health field. The same is true after a stroke or when one is diagnosed with diabetes—we focus on movement and exercise. But many people are not aware of the role exercise plays in reducing cancer risk. Let's change that and take control of our cancer risk through exercise! We need a new perspective about its importance.

How Does Exercise Reduce Your Cancer Risk?

I don't want to give a whole immunology lesson, but I do want to show you the various, scientifically validated ways that exercise helps prevent cancer. I'd like you to see that exercise helps with more than just your overall health—exercise creates changes in your body that help it to fight cancer (see Figure 7).

EFFECTS OF EXERCISE ON THE BODY

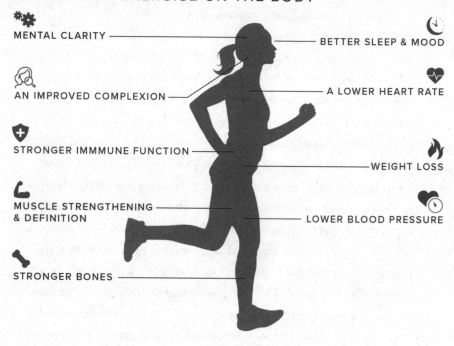

MENTAL CLARITY

BETTER SLEEP & MOOD

AN IMPROVED COMPLEXION

A LOWER HEART RATE

STRONGER IMMMUNE FUNCTION

WEIGHT LOSS

MUSCLE STRENGTHENING
& DEFINITION

LOWER BLOOD PRESSURE

STRONGER BONES

Figure 7

Exercise helps create healthier blood vessels. You may think you are building your biceps—and you are—but you are also exercising your arteries. When you are physically active, your heart rate goes up for a period. You might even measure your heart rate with different apps to "get in the zone." Exercise also causes your blood pressure to go up briefly. The increased heart rate and blood pressure help force blood through your arteries, making them wider and more flexible—a sign of healthy arteries. This flexibility is critical since, as we get older, our blood vessels start to get stiff. It's the stiffness that prevents our blood vessels from functioning well—just as the stiffness in our joints can make it more difficult for us to do certain tasks. The stretching of the vessels also releases chemicals that promote the creation of healthier blood vessels, such as capillaries.

Imagine running water through a hose at full strength. The hose expands to contain the strong flow. Same effect on your blood vessels. This change in blood flow not only prevents plaques from forming, but also helps maintain good blood flow throughout the body, which might prevent cancer cells from growing. This increased blood flow can deliver immune and cancer-fighting cells to an area where cancer is growing. (It may also help when people with cancer are receiving chemotherapy—helping the drugs get to the right place!) Exercise can impact the formation of new blood vessels, a process called angiogenesis. Usually that's a good thing—except when it comes to cancer cells. In that circumstance, you want to prevent cancer cells from getting the blood supply that allows them to grow. Cancer often accelerates angiogenesis, promoting cancer cell growth. By exercise moderating this overproduction of angiogenesis and reducing inflammation, it helps prevent cancer cells from getting their own blood supply, decreasing their ability to grow and causing them to have a premature death. It's how some chemotherapy treatments work!

Exercise causes an increase in adrenaline. You all know that feeling you get when you are "pumped up" and ready to fight if need be! If you go for a run, how do you feel afterward? Tired or invigorated? I bet invigorated! That's the adrenaline your body releases during exercise. Some data suggests these short bursts of adrenaline inhibit the growth of cancer cells. They may do this by empowering our "natural killer" cells, which are part of the body's immune response. They invade the tumor cells and prevent them from growing. Sometimes, they make the cancer cells burst and die. This is a critical defense and anti-cancer strategy because cancer cells often find ways to evade the body's anti-growth defenses. Just remember that longer bursts of adrenaline, usually associated with stress, likely do the opposite—promoting cancer growth.

Exercise contributes to weight loss. We know that obesity is related to several types of cancer, so anything that helps us lose excess fat can help reduce the risk of cancer. Exercise plays a key role in helping you burn more fat and calories, which typically leads to weight loss. It's a little more complicated than that since physical activity lowers your risk of cancer regardless of your weight or size.

Excess body fat causes multiple health problems. Don't think that fat is just "hanging" on your body, because it's doing much more. There's the fat that you can feel and pinch. But what's even more concerning is the fat you can't see that surrounds your organs. Our fat is metabolically active, meaning it functions like an organ! Excess fat stimulates the release of cytokines (chemicals that cause inflammation), causing chronic inflammation, and disrupts the proper processing of hormones like insulin. Fat cells are secreting or interacting with hormones and chemicals—like insulin, leptin, and estrogen—and disrupting our body's normal hormonal balance. As a result, our pancreas pumps out even more hormones! Excess amounts of fat can make our body resistant to processing glucose correctly. This creates insulin resistance, and it's an indicator of inflammation.

It makes your body a bit of a mess! But exercise can help reduce fat and the subsequent insulin problems.

Let's discuss this a little further. You probably know how insulin relates to diabetes, but proteins like insulin also play a specific role in cancer. Insulin-like growth factors in the bloodstream stimulate cells to grow. This includes normal cells but also abnormal cells. When there's fast growth in cell production, it's easier to make mistakes. With fast cell production, some cells might not turn out so well, meaning they are cancer cells instead of normal cells. Some of the abnormal cells can even prevent the body's attempt to destroy them. That's partly what makes cancer so difficult to treat.

Here's one of the ways exercise helps prevent cancer—it lowers the amount of excess fat, it reduces inflammation, and it lowers the amount of insulin and the insulin-like growth factors in the blood. Scientists are looking at metformin—a drug commonly prescribed for diabetes—as a possible medicine for cancer prevention, primarily because of its effect on reducing insulin resistance, and it effects on weight loss. If your body demonstrates insulin resistance—common in pre-diabetes and diabetes—your pancreas keeps pumping out more and more insulin than you typically need because your muscles and cells aren't responding to it as effectively as they did before. All this extra insulin starts to cause problems. Metformin makes the body more sensitive to the effects of insulin, so your pancreas doesn't keep pouring out hormones. In a way, it's duplicating through a pill what you can do through exercise.

Too much insulin resistance, the weight gain it causes, and the associated inflammation can lead to the production of too much estrogen. I mentioned earlier on that too much estrogen can be related to numerous cancers including post-menopausal breast cancer, ovarian cancer, and endometrial cancer. With estrogen, more is not better. The environment that has too much insulin and estrogen can accelerate cell production and being too fast can lead to errors. It's like rushing to bake five batches of cookies instead of two under a time deadline. Mistakes happen. When trying to prevent cancer, we need to try to keep our cell production machinery from making mistakes. Exercise's impact on weight loss and its effect on reducing excess hormones and inflammation is critical in your personal cancer prevention program.

Exercise promotes healthy digestion. Ever notice the impact of physical activity on your stomach as well as bowel habits? How does running impact your need "to go to the bathroom"? In medicine, we refer to it as bowel mobility. Physical activity reduces the time it takes for food to travel through the digestive system, which decreases the gastrointestinal (GI) tract organs' exposure to possible carcinogens. It also decreases the metabolism of bile acids and that makes more bile acid available and around in your body. Bile acids—which are needed to digest fats and fat-soluble vitamins—are thought to promote cancer cell progression if there are too many around. Some amount is necessary for our normal body function. Too many bile acids, however, seem to help cancer cells hide from our immune cells, which are trying to kill them. If we can lower the amount of bile acid production, we might be able to lower risk of some cancers such as colon cancer. Some of the strongest data supporting the role of exercise in cancer prevention comes from the treatment of colon cancer. I suspect that exercise's effect on the speed at which you digest and poop, and on the amount of bile acids you produce, are major reasons!

Exercise reduces chronic inflammation. Inflammation is good in the short term to help fight injury and infection. But like everything else, you can have too much of a good thing. Long-term inflammation damages your body and increases your risk for cancer by affecting how cells divide. Recent data suggests that just twenty minutes of daily exercise reduces inflammation in cells all over our body. Exercise reduces a substance called tumor necrosis factor (TNF) which uses inflammation to fight infection. The balance between high and low levels of TNF is complex, and when it comes to cancer development our body needs just the right amount. If you're healthy, your body naturally blocks any extra TNF you might have. But with an autoimmune disease like rheumatoid arthritis, for example, that doesn't happen, and you end up with too much TNF in your blood. That leads to inflammation and painful symptoms, typically in your joints, digestive tract, or skin, depending on what disease you have. The same unhealthy response occurs with cancer. Too much inflammation is going to cause damage to your cells' DNA, which promotes cancer cells. That's one of the reasons people with inflammatory bowel disease are at increased risk for colon cancer. Reducing inflammation through exercise is going to lower your cancer risk.

Exercise reduces stress. When I say stress, you are probably thinking of the way your body and mind feel when you are overscheduled, overworked, and overwhelmed. Exercise certainly helps reduce that stress. Answer this question for me: Have you ever felt bad after going to the gym? I bet you answered "no," especially if you've worked out after a stressful week. Exercise relieves psychological stress, partly by reducing stress hormones.

Exercise also helps with another type of stress called "oxidative stress." Our cells produce molecules called "free radicals." In theory, that sounds good—it's free and it's a radical! That might be good in politics, but it's not good when it comes to your body. Too many free radicals cause oxidative stress, which can damage your DNA. Exercise increases antioxidant activity, which helps to neutralize those free radicals, protecting you from cell damage and lowering your cancer risk.

I think most of us know that stress impacts our health. Keep in mind that it impacts your cancer risk too. Stress, whether physical or psychological, impacts the ability of your cells to grow and repair. That's why we need stress-combating therapies—like exercise—that reduce your odds of getting cancer.

Exercise directly strengthens our immune function through several mechanisms. It prevents cancer by directly activating and priming specific immune system defenders, including antibodies and white blood cells. These natural defenders destroy cancer cells and abnormal cells that could turn cancerous. Exercise also increases our body temperature. That's one of the reasons we sweat. This increased temperature provides an environment that allows immune cells to enter more easily into tumor cells and destroy them, as well as preventing poisonous cells from growing.

Cancer cells alter our metabolism, producing many more cancer cells, increasing their blood supply and escaping immune cells that try to destroy them. As a result, high lactate levels accumulate within tumors. These high levels may prevent our immune cells from functioning properly in getting their job done. Exercise lowers lactate and in theory may help prevent cancer cells from replicating.

Exercise changes the function and expression of our genes. We are just beginning to learn how exercise can activate or quiet certain genes. Imagine if we can turn on those genes that suppress cancer and turn off those genes that promote it! Exercise seems to be playing that sort of role, and that can be a huge benefit! Exercise may be changing our DNA structure as well as deciding how our genes work in expressing healthy or cancer cell growth. This is an exciting area of research that I think we will hear much more about in the next couple of years.

I hope I have convinced you that, although some of its mechanisms will be more important than others in preventing different types of cancer, exercise can help reduce your personal cancer risk in several ways. The great aspect about exercise is that it implements multiple strategies—it's a force multiplier. Your body might respond differently to exercise than my body—but its many benefits are the reason we should incorporate exercise as a component of our personal cancer prevention program.

An "Exercise Prescription"
for Cancer Prevention

I know that many doctors simply tell their patients, "You need to go to the gym." How often have you heard that? I have never found such a broad statement to be helpful, whether it's to reduce the risk of heart disease, diabetes, or cancer. The reduction in risk of cancer depends on the type of physical activity, the amount of effort, how long it lasts, as well as what type of cancer you are trying to prevent. We need specifics—not some general advice to "go work out." Some doctors are beginning to write "exercise prescriptions" with specific details to underscore its importance, but such prescriptions are still the exception. I've included an example of an exercise prescription for you at the end of this chapter.

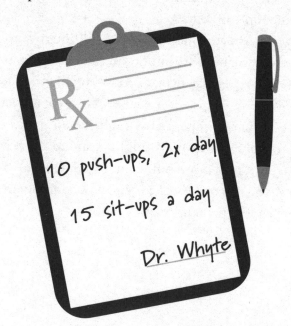

What Is "Exercise"?

Let's begin with the basics. What counts as exercise? Although we often use the terms "physical activity" and "exercise" interchangeably, they do have different meanings. Physical activity is any movement requiring energy to be carried out by the skeletal muscles. In other words, any movement you do is technically considered physical activity. Exercise, on the other hand, is planned, structured, repetitive, and intentional movement typically performed to improve or maintain physical fitness.

Drawing the distinction between the two terms really does matter. The term "exercise" is central when talking about cancer prevention. Here's why. When I say "exercise," many people are intimidated. They don't want to go to the gym either because of time, expense, or just embarrassment. I have had many patients over the years tell me they needed to get into shape before they could go to the gym!

But I've noticed that if I ask patients if they're being "physically active" I get a very different response. I've had people tell me they are very active, since they walk around at work or are busy with their kids. (I have two young boys and I am active with them, but I still seem to gain weight if I don't exercise!) They seem to think all this activity counts as exercise—but it doesn't! This activity is helpful for your overall health, but when it comes to cancer prevention, effort and exertion is key. "Exercise" is important because we create a routine or structure that is focused on improving health. It requires exertion, which allows you to get the benefits of becoming healthier and stronger. Simply going about your daily living, or walking from your desk to the printer, isn't going to provide the protection against cancer that exercise can. My cancer doctor friends like to say "sitting is the new smoking"—so we need to get you moving! The more you sit, the more you need to focus on exercise.

For cancer prevention, the American Cancer Society now recommends 150 to 300 minutes of moderate-intensity or 75 to 150 minutes of vigorous physical activity (or a combination of the two) every week (we'll go into exactly what "moderate" and "vigorous" mean a little further down). These guidelines, updated in 2020, recommend an increase in frequency and intensity based on data showing that exercise prevents cancer. I've seen that when people hear those numbers they find them daunting—and undoable! Three hundred minutes seems too much, doesn't it? I'm going to try to convince you that it's doable. Let's break it down.

In terms of moderate activity, that's about two and a half to five hours a week. Here's a better way to think about it: about twenty-five minutes a day of moderate exercise and fifteen minutes a day of vigorous exercise. That seems more doable, doesn't it? I have learned over the years that you need to schedule exercise—if you think you will "work in" working out, you're doomed to failure. It's what happened to me until I made exercise a priority. Just like sleep, your exercise time seems to be the first thing to go when your day gets busy. That is why you need to make a weekly plan of how and when you will exercise. Even if you can't do that much at once, don't give up. Sometimes you need to "sneak it in" during the day—ten minutes here, twenty minutes there. Go slow and gradually build up time. Some exercise is better than none.

The good news, however, is that more is better. Although we need more research on the optimal dose, as well as type and intensity, we do know that moderate to high-intensity exercise is better than light exercise. There seems to be a linear relationship between the amount of exercise a person gets and cancer risk, particularly for breast and colon cancer. Meaning, the more exercise you do, the more benefits you get and the lower your risk.

Can you exercise too much? Doctors used to think that too much exercise could weaken your immune system. A recent analysis showed that endurance sports can boost our body's ability to fight infection, sending white blood cells to key organs to help protect them. Of course, you need to be careful of overexertion and injuries, but most of us aren't going to need to worry about exercising too much.

Moderate Activity

What's moderate activity? There are lots of different definitions, but mine is simple. Moderate-intensity activity should get your heart rate to 50 to 70 precent of your maximum heart rate. Your maximum heart rate is 220 minus your age.

For most people, examples include swimming, bicycling about 12 miles per hour (no big hills!), or walking at a pace of about 3.5 miles an hour (see Figure 8).

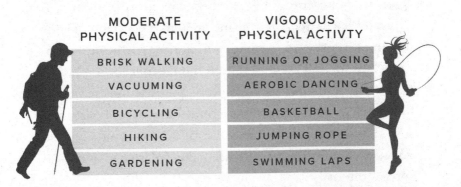

MODERATE PHYSICAL ACTIVITY	VIGOROUS PHYSICAL ACTIVTY
BRISK WALKING	RUNNING OR JOGGING
VACUUMING	AEROBIC DANCING
BICYCLING	BASKETBALL
HIKING	JUMPING ROPE
GARDENING	SWIMMING LAPS

Figure 8

What doesn't count? You can't base activity intensity on time alone. A leisurely walk for thirty minutes probably doesn't qualify as moderate activity for most people. Check your heart rate to make sure you are exerting yourself. What about using your steps as a measure of exercise? My advice is not to rely solely on the number of steps. I have plenty of patients who tell me they average about ten thousand steps a day. That sounds great when you first consider it, but if you are not exerting yourself with an elevated heart rate for at least twenty minutes, you aren't meeting your cancer prevention goal. You are helping with other aspects of your health but not directly impacting your cancer risk.

In addition, being busy at work or at home doesn't count either. "I'm running around all the time" is a response I often get when I talk to patients about exercise. I know it seems like you are running around, but in their everyday lives most people are just not running around with enough intensity to benefit.

Vigorous Activity

What's vigorous exercise? Most of us probably think we are vigorously exercising, but the reality is most of us aren't. Typically, it's defined as working at 70 to 85 percent of your maximal heart rate. Activities including running, swimming laps, biking at more than ten miles per hour, playing basketball, and jumping rope. Remember, some medicines for blood pressure and other conditions affect heart rate, so it's always good to check with your doctor about exercise goals, particularly when you are using heart rate as a measure of intensity.

Many activities can be moderate or vigorous depending upon your exertion. How do you differentiate between moderate and vigorous? I have a few suggestions. A variety of tracker apps are available for your smartphone. We've come a long way from when we only had pedometers! You could also use fitness bands and watches. In general, they are pretty good. They have become much more accurate in recent years, they're pretty durable and lightweight, and if you keep them on most of the time, you really don't even realize they are there, collecting lots of useful data. I used one for quite some time after noticing that my weight was going up as my age was going up! I saw the association between my lack of exercise and my weight going up. I needed the feedback and the trends analysis to keep me on the right track. It also was a rude awakening. The trackers showed me I wasn't burning the calories that I thought I was some days. I adjusted my behavior, and I found it motivating. It encouraged me to do more. They're not for everyone, but, especially early on, they can give you data about how your body is responding to exercise. On the other hand, I'm not a big fan of those monitors that are built into gym equipment, such as ellipticals. They're just not as precise as people think they are and may give you inaccurate information.

Another way to estimate exercise intensity without any special equipment: the talk test. To perform the talk test, see if you can talk or sing while performing the activity. If you're exercising moderately, you should be able to talk, but not sing. If you're exercising vigorously, you shouldn't be able to say more than a few words. It's not the time to be a "chatty Cathy," especially if you're part of a group activity.

A good friend relates that the instructor of her water aerobics class told the group that if they could carry on a conversation, they weren't working hard enough. Some of the ladies, who loved socializing during class, did not appreciate being called out! I also like this test because we all have gone to the gym at some point, ended up talking to friends more than exercising, imagined we "spent an hour" at the gym, and wondered why we don't see benefits! It's happened to me.

How Do You Get Started?

So now you know what to do, but how do you get started? Most people are able to exercise, but it's a good idea to talk to your doctor before you start, especially if you haven't been active for a long time, or if you have several health conditions. I know that creating an exercise routine can be intimidating, so it's a good idea to get some instruction. You might want to use an in-person or virtual personal trainer for a few sessions. Apps also can be very useful for helping you figure out how to get started and stay interested. There are even some personalized workout algorithms driven by artificial intelligence that help guide a truly personalized routine. I always encourage instruction, because so many people perform exercises incorrectly. When your form is faulty, you risk injury, especially as you get older. More important, if you are doing it wrong, you are just wasting time. Many of us simply do cardio since it seems easy to do, right? How hard is it to jump on a machine and pedal? But for cancer prevention, the data shows that cardio alone is not sufficient.

I know many of you associate exercise with going to a gym, which can be a turnoff. It requires time; it can be expensive, and even embarrassing. Frankly, it scares some people. I mentioned at the beginning of the chapter the remark that I've heard from many patients over the years: "I need to get in shape first." Some of us use the gym as a place for social gathering instead of focusing on sweat and health. If gyms stress you out—for whatever reason—then don't use them. Work out at home instead. Keep in mind that the key to successful exercise is to reach some level of exertion, and you soon realize it doesn't really matter where you do it.

I don't want you to get bogged down by different terms. Aerobic versus anerobic. Cardio versus resistance. Muscle strengthening versus balancing. It's a whole new vocabulary and it can be distracting. Don't worry about all that if you are just starting out. Simply focus on moving and exerting yourself. And be sure to mix in various types of exercises. I can help you learn these terms because they do have some importance, but for now you just need to start and do something. Don't overthink it. You want to develop new habits that include exercise. We used to think it takes twenty-one days to form a habit, but it may actually take sixty days or longer.

The great news is that there are many different types of exercise nowadays. You need to pick the ones that you enjoy because those are what you will stick with. If you don't like putting your head under water, don't choose swimming because you know it's a good form of exercise! That simply won't last long term. Whatever exercise you choose, start slow, take your time, and incorporate more exercises as you go along. I also suggest you consider using some type of journal or logbook early on. We tend to forget what we do: "Did I do thirty minutes or forty-five minutes on the elliptical? Was that ten reps or twelve?" You will make progress easier if you track what you are doing for a while.

When it comes to cancer prevention, strength training is important (see Figure 9). Researchers at the University of Sydney studied nearly eighty thousand adults and found that strength training, done twice a week, reduced the likelihood of dying from cancer by 31 percent. That shouldn't surprise you—we just went over the ways that exercise helps to prevent cancer: reversing the impact of obesity on our cells' ability to process insulin and making our body more sensitive to insulin, rather than resistant! If participants added cardio workouts, the risk of dying from cancer decreased even more. Cardio alone did not have much of an effect on cancer death. Remember, strength training doesn't have to mean buying weights and going to the gym. Push-ups, squats, crunches, lunges—the dreaded plank!—all count as strength training and can be done basically anywhere. Don't forget about yoga either!

For many people, the psychological aspect of starting and maintaining a regular exercise program can pose a hurdle. Maybe you think of it as a chore—or even a punishment. Sometimes I wish we didn't call it "working out"—since that makes it seem like work! Instead, try to reframe exercise as a gift to yourself, a habit you want to create. You aren't "spending" time working out—you are investing time in yourself. And it's an investment you won't regret: a consistent exercise habit will not only lower your cancer risk, but also protect your heart and provide all those other health benefits I mentioned at the beginning of the chapter.

REDUCTION OF CANCER THROUGH EXERCISE

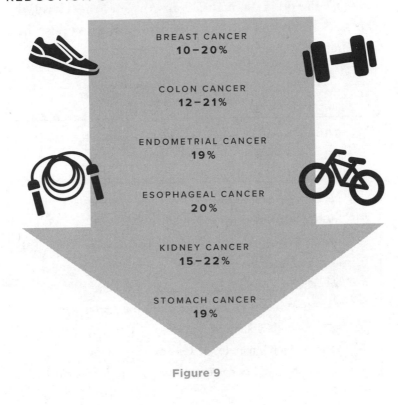

BREAST CANCER
10–20%

COLON CANCER
12–21%

ENDOMETRIAL CANCER
19%

ESOPHAGEAL CANCER
20%

KIDNEY CANCER
15–22%

STOMACH CANCER
19%

Figure 9

Summary

Exercise is a powerful tool to prevent cancer. It blocks cancer cells from forming and growing, and helps the body fight cancer. But remember, your typical daily activities are not sufficiently intense to provide the health benefits you want. To get the maximum benefit from exercise, consistency, exertion (with elevated heart rate), and variety are key. You need to create a plan to incorporate cardio and strength training on most days of the week. I bet you'll be amazed at how your body—and your life—will transform.

Exercise can't eliminate cancer risk completely, but it can decrease the odds. No matter your current fitness level, you can benefit right now from incorporating exercise into your personal cancer prevention program.

ANSWERS

1. **TRUE**—Exercise has been shown to decrease the risk of several cancers.

2. **FALSE**—Cardio alone does not provide the cancer-prevention benefits of exercise. You need to incorporate resistance training.

3. **FALSE**—Exercise's effect on cancer prevention is not limited to people who are overweight. It has numerous benefits for people regardless of their weight.

4. **FALSE**—There is no data to suggest that too much exercise hurts your immune system.

5. **TRUE**—Twenty minutes of daily exercise, done consistently, has been demonstrated to reduce the risk of cancer.

CHAPTER SEVEN

Is There a Mind-Body Connection?

TRUE OR FALSE?

1. If you actively think you won't get cancer, then you won't.
2. People who are depressed have a higher rate of cancer.
3. The science behind a mind-body connection is only a few decades old.
4. Stress can make cancer cells grow.
5. Practicing mindfulness can make your immune system stronger.

(Answers at end of chapter)

GOING THROUGH MEDICAL SCHOOL, I never really understood the mind-body connection. It simply wasn't taught back then, and the people who espoused it were not considered mainstream. If you wanted to get ahead in the medical world, talking about the mind's connection to the body wasn't going to get you far, even though the role of emotions in health has been recognized for thousands of years.

Then I met Dr. Dean Ornish, who talked about diet as a way to prevent heart attacks but also discussed the importance of stress management and relationships as treatment. He was asking how much love and support you have. What?? He's asking about *love* as well as cholesterol? Whoa! No one was talking about that in the '80s and '90s!

Fast-forward twenty years—we now readily acknowledge that the mind impacts the body. In fact, the connection is mainstream science—unlike when I started my medical training. Dr. Ornish and other researchers helped change our understanding of the mind-body connection by publishing clinical studies that showed the role that stress reduction and social connections have in reducing plaque and, consequently, heart attacks. The benefits aren't limited to the heart. If stress reduction prevents heart disease, it makes sense that it would reduce the incidence of other diseases too. Dr. Ornish has started to do the same type of work in cancer, particularly prostate cancer.

It's surprising that it took so long for us in the medical field to acknowledge the mind-body connection, because there's really no doubt that our mind—particularly our thoughts, feelings, and attitudes—affects how our body functions. And it does so in good ways but also bad ways.

Think about it—when you are happy, you feel like you can accomplish anything. You climb a hill as a kid and proclaim yourself "king of the world." During moments of excitement and joy, you can feel your heart racing. My young son likes to say his "heart smiles" when he gets excited. I can quickly learn a lot about a patient's condition simply by looking at him or her. I always tell patients that if you can laugh while you're talking to me, it's unlikely you are having a heart attack.

When you are sad, how does your body feel? Tired? Achy? I bet you feel lousy all over. When you get angry or frustrated, you might get a headache or even feel dizzy. Or when someone is annoying you, you can feel your blood pressure going up—and if you measure it, you see that it does! What do you experience before a big presentation? Sweaty palms and nervousness!

I suspect you can tell when you are stressed. Does your stomach feel like it's churning? Or maybe you start having diarrhea? You might feel restless or experience rapid breathing. These are all examples of your emotions affecting your body—in ways you can directly feel. Our minds and bodies are definitely connected. We make the connection between the mind and the body during these short moments that I described! It makes sense, then, that our feelings and emotions have a long-term impact, too, on our bodies.

Stress is a prime example. We know that the stress of our jobs and working long hours does more than just make us feel "stressed"—it has a major influence on our health (see Figure 10). A recent study in the medical journal *Lancet* found that people working fifty-five or more hours per week had a 33 percent increased risk of stroke and a 13 percent greater risk of developing heart disease compared to people who worked less than forty hours a week. Studies also show that chronic stress and exhaustion can play a role in the development of atrial fibrillation—an abnormal heart rhythm that can cause health problems. Doesn't it make sense that our feelings and emotions can also impact other parts of our body—including the ability to fight cancer?

EFFECTS OF CHRONIC STRESS

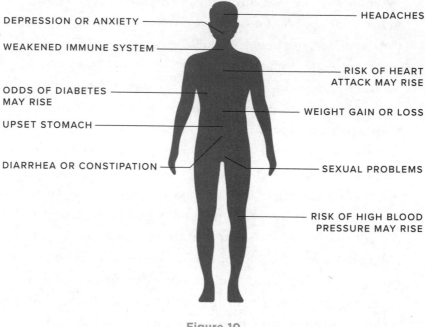

DEPRESSION OR ANXIETY

WEAKENED IMMUNE SYSTEM

ODDS OF DIABETES
MAY RISE

UPSET STOMACH

DIARRHEA OR CONSTIPATION

HEADACHES

RISK OF HEART
ATTACK MAY RISE

WEIGHT GAIN OR LOSS

SEXUAL PROBLEMS

RISK OF HIGH BLOOD
PRESSURE MAY RISE

Figure 10

Keep in mind that short periods of stress do not cause problems in our immune system. Short periods of stress have an immune-building result. The best example of good stress is our fight-or-flight response. You want to summon stress hormones to make you more alert, ready to respond to a potentially life-threatening event. We need that stress to survive! It's chronic stress that causes the problems.

Sometimes we forget that the workings of our minds are conscious and unconscious. Our mind-body connection is not always so obvious. Sometimes you can feel the effect—like that queasy stomach—and sometimes you aren't aware of the impact and damage until much later. We have emotional reactions that lead to physical effects—and many times we don't connect our physical pain to our emotional and mental health. For example, we know that depression can cause physical pain—but still we tend to miss the connection when it comes to our personal situation. Sometimes we can see it in others, but not ourselves.

How Does This Mind-Body Connection Affect Your Cancer Risk?

The health of our minds definitely affects our immunity, and chronic stress may increase cancer risk both directly and indirectly. Stress hormones can inhibit a process called anoikis—meaning "without a home"—which kills cancer cells and stops them from spreading. The tumor cells have nowhere to live and ultimately die as a result. Some data suggests that stress can play a role in shortening telomeres, which are basically caps at the end of our DNA. Some people describe them as bumpers protecting our cells. When these get shorter, our DNA becomes more vulnerable to damage, and that affects our overall health, including cancer risk. Ongoing chronic stress also increases the production of certain growth factors that increase your blood supply. This can help cancer grow and spread. There is some early data that suggests elevated levels of norepinephrine could possibly cause cancer cells that previously were "quiet" to awaken and start growing and spreading again. We also know that stress impacts our sleep as well as our weight—both of which affect the risk of cancer. Stress also increases our use of substances, such as alcohol, illicit drugs, and tobacco, which we often use in an attempt to blunt the feelings of stress, yet also raise your odds of certain cancers.

Stress isn't the only player in the mind-body connection. Our emotions—especially if chronic—like anger, fear, guilt, jealousy, anxiety, resentment, and sadness manifest in the body in different ways—sometimes leading to disease. Repressed emotions are especially harmful. These emotions and thoughts change the way the body functions at hormonal, cellular, and immunologic levels, thereby increasing your risk of disease, including cancer.

Let me be clear. Your mental and physical health are complex and connected. This connection contributes to determining your personal cancer risk. If you want to decrease your odds of getting cancer, you need to manage both.

For instance, many scientists believe there is a biological relationship between depression and some cancers. It's easy to think that if you have cancer, you are likely to develop depression and perhaps other mental health issues. But your mental health, itself, can increase your odds of a cancer diagnosis.

We know that depressed people have a higher mortality rate than people who are not depressed. That rate includes death from conditions other than cancer, but numerous studies have shown that people who are depressed have higher rates of cancer, particularly breast cancer and prostate cancer. Some data also shows a connection between bipolar disease and brain cancer.

A study done a few years ago in the UK found that men over forty who suffer from generalized anxiety disorder are more than twice as likely to die of cancer than are men who do not have an anxiety disorder. What I find fascinating is that even after researchers took account of factors that increase the risk of cancer, including age, alcohol consumption, smoking, and chronic diseases, men with a diagnosis of generalized anxiety disorder were still more likely to die of cancer. These findings were not observed in the women they studied. I don't want you to think that you can worry yourself into a cancer diagnosis, but anxiety does affect your immune system, so it is critical you don't ignore it.

Ever hear of broken heart syndrome? Losing a loved one is emotionally devastating but it's also physical damaging. Psychological stress triggers weakening of heart muscles, which can cause shortness of breath and chest tightness. We all have seen stories where elderly couples who have spent their lives together often die within days or months of each other. Our emotions affect our physical health!

Just as our emotions have a powerful effect on our bodies, so do our thoughts and attitudes. Attitude matters. A growing body of evidence demonstrates that people who have a positive outlook on life, who are optimistic, are less likely to become sick. Middle-aged adults who are more optimistic about their future tend to have higher serum antioxidant levels than their less optimistic peers. These antioxidants help reduce cancer cell activity. Research has shown that people who are cynical have a greater risk of dementia and heart disease compared to those who are more trusting and optimistic.

Tell me, would you consider yourself friendly or more standoffish? I ask because some research suggests that people who score higher on measures of unfriendliness, as well as those with chronic stress and depressive symptoms, have a higher risk of stroke and transient ischemic attacks than the friendlier, kinder participants. It could be due to the activation of harmful hormonal pathways that weaken our immune system.

Whether we live with clinical depression, harbor repressed negative emotions, or simply have a sour attitude, our negative emotions and thoughts impact our overall health and can also affect our risk of getting cancer. When you are angry and have negative emotions, you tend not to socialize or connect with others, right? "Sometimes, I just want to stay home and brood for a while," one patient is fond of telling me. I also have a friend who says she "keeps a list"—I hope just a mental one!—of the slights she has experienced from relatives and friends. She avoids those who have "wronged" her. There's a Buddhist saying: "Anger is like a poison that you drink yourself, but you think will hurt the other person."

If you experience depression or anxiety, you might have difficulty reaching out for connection because you feel isolated. You may not have the energy to interact with relatives, friends, or even coworkers. When we are cut off from social connections, for whatever reason, we miss out on the mental and physical benefits that could help lower our cancer risk.

Negative emotions can take another indirect toll on us, through the lifestyle habits they often bring along. They likely impact your sleep, eating habits, and willingness to exercise. When you are stressed or depressed or angry, you might overeat as well as consume more alcohol. I have a patient who, despite my urging to quit smoking, always tells me "smoking calms my nerves." It can be an unhealthy cycle in which your struggle with stressful emotions is coupled with habits that further decrease the body's immune response. To top it off, if you are struggling with negative emotions or an untreated mental health condition, you might not feel motivated to stay on top of your health care. You might skip cancer screenings or might be less likely to take quick action if early cancer symptoms surface (or you may not even notice them).

A good friend of mine often compares checking his mental health to checking his car. He remarks that he wishes we had a "low oil light" for emotions and feelings. That way, we would know we need to tend to them. Too often, we simply aren't aware of what's going on. If we don't check our mental health, we'll have the same problem we have when we don't check our oil: we aren't going to get very far, and there can be major problems.

The good news is it's never too late to change. Addressing unproductive, negative, and harmful thoughts, emotions, and feelings can improve your health. Neural pathways are constantly changing—a concept known as "neuroplasticity." Consider this as a new motto: change your thoughts, change your brain, change your health, change your cancer risk.

Maximizing the Mind-Body Connection

So, how you do use the mind-body connection as part of your personal cancer prevention program?

Take stress seriously. No one expects you to be a superhero. It's important to understand the negative consequences of stress, especially when it comes to your cancer risks. Chronic stress is not something anyone in our society should take lightly. Do not assume stress will simply go away or that somehow it won't affect you as it does others or that you can outsmart its effects, because you can't. Now is the time to reduce stress in your life; not add to it.

Build a stress-management toolbox. There are going to be times when you cannot get rid of stress. That's just the reality of life. You're going to have to manage it, just as you do other health conditions. Try to identify your sources of stress. You likely know what they are. Can they be changed in any way? Even if you can't rid yourself of the source of your stress, you might be able to modify it. Many experts suggest "microsteps"—small changes over time that can help restore resilience. It might be learning to say "no" to things and scaling back on your commitments. Or it might mean doing something big, like a career or relationship change. Money is often a big stressor, and you might need to change how you spend money and what you spend it on. Not everyone can afford a financial advisor, and managing money can be confusing. Luckily, there a lot of good, credible, free online resources to help with some of your money questions and planning.

This toolbox can help you keep a lid on chronic stress. It also can help you prevent minor sources of stress from lingering to a point where they're affecting your health.

Identify emotions and thoughts that are having a negative impact on your health. Call it what it is. To address your emotions, you need to acknowledge them. Name what you are feeling—whether it's fear, sadness, jealousy, anxiety, or anger—with no apology or judgment. Once you acknowledge your feelings, you can then start to address them. It's truly the first step.

Practice forgiveness. For many of us it's difficult to forgive, isn't it? We were wronged and we aren't going to forget it, right? Fool me once, shame on you. Fool me twice, shame on me! Are you the type of person that holds a grudge? We all know people—especially in our families—who still are mad about something that happened at a wedding twenty-five years ago! This mindset creates problems. There are some doctors who suggest unforgiveness should be considered a disease. Within the past few years, we have seen numerous studies demonstrate that forgiveness lowers the risk of heart attack, improves lipid profile, improves sleep, and reduces pain. If you want to improve your health, you are going to need to forgive.

Try mindfulness to address unhealthy thoughts and emotions. What image comes into your mind when I first say "mindfulness"? For many years, I immediately pictured a group of monks sitting on a dirt floor chanting "om." I simply didn't know enough about it, and quite frankly didn't understand it. I had to overcome a bias I had against it since it didn't seem part of "mainstream medicine."

The practice of mindfulness is thousands of years old. The concept of mindfulness comes from ancient Buddhism, although our current versions of mindfulness are more secular, without any focus on religion. Several hundred medical centers around the world offer mindfulness programs to promote health, especially as it relates to anxiety and mood disorders. Numerous studies have shown that the practice of mindfulness can change the structure of some areas of your brain, especially those that are involved in emotions.

Usually starting with deep focus on the breath, a mindful person pays full attention to the present moment, and simply notices, without judgment, all the thoughts, feelings, and sensations associated with that moment. There should be no emotional reaction.

We've seen the benefits of mindfulness in people that have cancer. Researchers have shown that practicing mindfulness has a positive impact at the cellular level in patients with breast cancer. It also seems to impact those telomeres I mentioned earlier. These practices can also release neurotransmitters, such as dopamine, serotonin, melatonin, and epinephrine, that impact our physical and mental health, especially anxiety. In addition, it likely reduces cortisol levels. Researchers are also studying whether it decreases interleukin-6, a protein that promotes a state of chronic inflammation, making it hard for the immune system to function properly.

You may be wondering if mindfulness and meditation are the same thing. They have similarities but also some differences. Some experts will compare them this way: mindfulness is the awareness of "some-thing," while meditation is the awareness of "no-thing." Think of it this way: the aim of mindfulness is to bring your awareness to the present moment, whether you are sitting quietly, running errands, gardening, cooking, or walking the dog. Whatever you are doing, you are being conscious of the experience. Meditation is more active; you aren't just being aware of the present moment, but you are trying to bring your attention to a specific point of focus. Some studies of monks show meditation-related changes in different areas of the brain—particularly growth in those areas that process sensory information! The difference is between paying attention (mindfulness) and directing attention (meditation). Both can play a role in your personal cancer prevention program to reduce your cancer risk. Give them a try and see which might be best for you.

I often recommend patients to look online or try some apps to make sure they are practicing mindfulness or meditation correctly. You can't just go in a room and turn off the lights. It does take some practice to get the most benefits. Don't give up after just a few times but rather make a commitment to do it at least for a month, and then see how you feel. If you want the benefits, you need to engage in regular practice of meditation—just like for exercise and healthy eating. Mastering the mind can help you master the body. Why not give it a try?

Breathing is key. Of course, we need to breathe to live. But how we breathe at times affects our mental health. Consider trying "box breathing." It's a four-part cycle of four seconds each. You breathe in, hold in, breathe out, hold out. By focusing on your breathing in and out, you reduce your anxiety over time. I know it seems hard to believe that things this simple can work, but there's good evidence to show focused breathing can help with our mental health. Surely you have sixteen seconds every day to try this!

Schedule gratitude. We can get caught up in what we are unhappy with in our lives, and take for granted many of the positive things. One patient described the gratitude reminders she gives herself when she feels particularly stressed or sad. She sets a daily alarm and when it goes off she takes a couple minutes to reflect on what she is thankful for. "Sometimes it's about things not happening to me—like not being out of work, not being alone, not being hungry. Other times it's the joy I experience in seeing my grandchildren and being able to travel. I stopped comparing myself to others a long time ago." Gratitude helps you change your focus to what you have versus what you lack. A few years ago, a family member encouraged me to do a "gratitude note" every day for a month. After the first couple of days, you really begin to think about what matters. It can make a big difference.

Give biofeedback a try. Biofeedback is another strategy that can help weaken the links between the unhealthy thoughts and emotions that lead to unhealthy physical responses. Biofeedback harnesses the power of your mind and awareness of what's going on inside your body to give you more control over your health. It's been used to treat conditions such as chronic pain and urinary incontinence, manage pain without medication, and ease daily headaches. It's also been helpful in the management of chronic stress and emotional discomfort. You watch how your body responds as you change your heart rate, blood pressure, and breathing. By recognizing emotional triggers and cues, and the physiologic response they generate, you can help control how your mind and body respond.

Make sure you laugh. Do you laugh much? If you don't, try to! Research shows laughter decreases stress hormones, increases HDL cholesterol (the "good" cholesterol), and reduces artery inflammation. There's even some data that suggests it increases the immunoglobulins in our saliva that protect our respiratory tract. Laughter also releases endorphins—those "feel-good" hormones. It also strengthens our immune system, increasing the number of antibodies in our blood and white blood cells that fight infection in addition to improving blood flow. And who doesn't enjoy a good chuckle? It definitely changes your mood.

Researchers suggest that smiling—even if you aren't happy—can trick your brain into feeling happiness. The act of smiling can release neurotransmitters that act as antidepressants. Our facial expressions affect our emotional feelings. Granted, you can't actually smile your way to happiness, but you can make changes to how you are feeling based on your expressions.

Savor pleasure. Sometimes we just need to slow down and enjoy what's around us. Perhaps it's eating slowly, enjoying the flavor of a well-cooked meal, or watching a beautiful sunset. Taking some time every now and then to read a good book or enjoy a movie. You might even treat yourself to a spa appointment! The key is to feel pleasure, which will maximize both your emotional and physical health.

Control what you can and try to let the rest go. You are not going to be able to change what other people do, no matter how hard you try. But you can control what you do and how you respond. Stop trying to change other people, and instead focus on how you can make your life better. Be sure to take care of your physical needs. This means trying to eat healthy, getting in some daily exercise, and sleeping seven to eight hours a night. Remember, the mind-body connection works both ways. You can't eat junk food and sit around all day and think your mental health and emotions won't suffer.

Get support. When emotions and stress get overwhelming— when you find it hard to manage your day—it might be time to talk to a professional. Too often in the past, there was a potentially harmful "pull yourself up by your own bootstraps" mindset. That's not an effective strategy to help promote mental wellness. Asking for help is an important step. A psychiatrist or psychologist can help teach you healthy ways to manage your stress. Strategy options may include talk therapy, medication, or cognitive behavioral therapy (CBT).

————

Summary

It's time we all recognize the mind-body relationship as part of a personal cancer prevention program. The mind and body are inseparable. Healthy minds equal healthy bodies. Remember this: there's no physical health without mental health. They share a common biological and chemical language; they speak to and affect each other. We are still learning how our emotions, mindset, and attitude directly impact cancer risk. But we do know that one of the best things you can do for your body is to tend to your mind. You will not only lower your cancer risk; you will be happier too.

ANSWERS

1. **FALSE**—Cancer is determined by several factors. Although the health of your mind affects the health of your body and can reduce cancer risk, you can't think cancer away.

2. **TRUE**—People with depression do have greater risk of cancer.

3. **FALSE**—The science is thousands of years old.

4. **TRUE**—Stress can make cancer cells grow.

5. **TRUE**—Mindfulness can strengthen the immune system.

CHAPTER EIGHT

Can Restorative Sleep Help Prevent Cancer?

TRUE OR FALSE?

1. You need less sleep as you get older.
2. Working at night increases your risk of certain types of cancer.
3. Melatonin can prevent cancer.
4. Hitting the "snooze" button is okay as long as you don't do it every day.
5. Napping during the day can help you sleep better at night.

(Answers at end of chapter)

"HONESTLY, DOC, I DON'T HAVE time to sleep. My work commute is over an hour away, and by the time I get home, I still need to make dinner, take care of the kids, and catch up on housework. I will get around to it when I'm less busy." That was Angela's response when I told her she needed to sleep more than five hours a night. She was experiencing headaches, and she was always tired. Although she knew she was not sleeping enough, she wasn't associating her fatigue with her lack of restorative sleep. "Maybe I should get my thyroid checked?" she suggested at one point.

I completely understand Angela's reasoning. When you train to be a doctor, you give up a lot of sleep. During my residency, we had to stay up all night, every other night, for weeks at a time. No one complained because back then the department chair would quip, "The only problem with staying up every other night is that you miss half the cases." No one acknowledged the relationship between sleep—especially restorative sleep—and your overall health. Ironically, you would think that those who are teaching medicine to young doctors would recognize that adequate sleep is a critical factor for maximal health. Sadly, sleep wasn't considered something important—it was perceived as something getting in the way of work and learning. Honestly, it really wasn't until the last decade or so that we started to realize that our number of zzzs may correlate with our number of years.

Despite the overwhelming data about the importance of sleep, many people still don't think it's important for them. "I will sleep when I'm dead" is a refrain I have heard from many patients over the years. Sadly, it was often from people who had health issues and didn't see the relationship between their poor health and poor sleep. Others feel sleep is keeping them from "living life" when the reality is that good sleep over time helps them enjoy life. We have a "FOMO" (fear of missing out) mentality, and sleep gets in the way. By the end of this chapter, though, I hope to convince you that less sleep may mean less life.

Most of us don't spend much time thinking about our sleep and its effect on our health. After all, we sleep every day. And when we are busy, what's the first thing we cut back on? You got it—sleep! We always seem to think we will have plenty of time to sleep later. We view a restful night of sleep as a luxury rather than a necessity; yet, science shows that good sleep quality is as important as diet and exercise for maximum health. Some people like to brag about how much they accomplish with little sleep. "I only need four hours a night"—we all know some folks who say that. Some people still equate lack of sleep with a strong work ethic, even though inadequate sleep impacts our health and ultimately decreases work productivity. Sleep deprivation should not be used as a badge of honor. No one really feels good after an "all-nighter" no matter the reason—important job assignment, school task, or even newborn baby. It certainly is not a good approach when it comes to designing your personal cancer prevention strategy. Our brains do NOT adapt to less sleep. That's why the National Highway Traffic Safety Administration limits the amount of time that truckers can drive, without a mandated rest period. It's the same for pilots, mandated by the Federal Aviation Administration. The folks at Guinness World Records don't sanction sleep deprivation records anymore—it's considered too dangerous!

Sleep isn't just time for your brain to "turn off." In fact, your brain doesn't go into "sleep mode" like your computer. PET scans show many regions of our brain remain active while we sleep. If we stick with the computer analogy, think of sleep as the time your brain spends updating and consolidating your neural circuitry. Just as your computer and phone need time to periodically "update," so, too, does our body, or problems arise.

How do you feel when you don't get enough sleep? You're irritable, short-tempered, inattentive, and just not happy. That's because sleep regulates our emotions. It also helps consolidate our memories. It helps make our memories "stick" and be transferred from one area of the brain to another area. Didn't you always try to get a good night's sleep before an important test? Experts like to quip "you may make memories while awake, but you keep memories in your sleep." Poor sleep correlates with the probability of developing dementia.

As during exercise, the lymphatic system removes toxins from our body while we sleep. Sleep also affects our physical reflexes and fine motor skills. Too little sleep for just one night can make you feel impaired as if you were drunk. Your walking may be unstable, and your hand strength might be weakened. Would you want to have surgery done by someone who got just four hours of sleep the night before? I know I wouldn't. Why do we make sure athletes get a good night's sleep before a big game? It's not just so they can be alert and make good decisions; it's also to avoid injury. Lack of sleep decreases performance and increases the likelihood of injury. Is it a coincidence that the first year the Seattle Seahawks tracked and monitored sleep, they won the Super Bowl?!

Sleep is grow time! If you've ever seen your children in the morning and thought "it looks like they grew overnight," it's because they did. It's during deep sleep that children literally get bigger. Sleep sends a signal to our body to release growth hormones children need to develop.

For maximum health benefit, we need to be getting quality sleep, which leaves you waking refreshed. We know sleeping too little can cause health problems, but sleeping too much can also signal health issues. I always tell patients that problems with sleep may be a sign of a more serious health issue, and you need to tell your doctor if you are having problems with your sleep, especially if you have trouble falling asleep, maintaining sleep, or if you are simply waking up tired. I have had many patients whose poor sleep was a sign of thyroid disease, heart problems, depression, and undetected cancer.

Relationship of Sleep and Cancer

I know that it may seem difficult to believe that how much you sleep can play a role in the development of cancer, but we've learned that too little sleep, as well as too much sleep, predicts a shorter life. The seriousness of the relationship between sleep and cancer became apparent when researchers found that people who do shift work are at greater risk for cancer. Shift work typically refers to employment that is outside of the normal 8:00 a.m. to 6:00 p.m. work cycle. It often involves nights, weekends, early morning—typically done in rotating shifts. Shift work has been identified as a likely carcinogen by the World Health Organization because of its effect on sleep. Some countries have recognized this relationship. Medscape reported in 2009 that Denmark paid compensation to women who developed breast cancer after long shifts of night work.

Numerous studies have shown a significant relationship between sleep and cancer. For instance, men who sleep only three to five hours a night have a more than 50 percent increased risk of developing prostate cancer, and people who get no more than six hours of sleep a night are at greater risk of colorectal cancer.

Considering the huge role sleep plays in our life—as much as one-third of it—it should be an important component of your personal cancer prevention program. When we recognize that sleep is more than just rest, we start to realize its importance. In a way, it's kind of strange that sleep is something that everyone does every day of our lives, yet we are just beginning to learn more about it.

Let's take a look at what we know about sleep and cancer risk.

Circadian Rhythm

To understand sleep, you need to understand your circadian rhythm cycle—the twenty-four-hour daily rhythm that governs so many of your bodily processes (see Figure 11). Some people refer to it as your "master clock." Circadian rhythm controls nearly every biological system in your body. This rhythm regulates certain hormone production as well as how some cells grow, repair, function, and even die. It controls your body temperature and whether or not you are hungry. When we have trouble sleeping, it's usually a result of some disruption to that cycle. I bet you've noticed you feel "different" for a few days when you travel to different time zones. Your body clock and the new environment aren't quite synced up and your body and brain get confused. That's your circadian rhythm out of whack. Imagine how that can impact you if it is occurring every day.

Circadian rhythm is impacted by several factors—especially light. So it's no coincidence that light is one of the biggest disruptors to your sleep. Light is good, except when it's at the wrong time of day. Why? Circadian rhythm is set up so that when it starts to get dark, we naturally start to shut down and sleep. If we experience light when we normally would experience darkness, it makes our rhythm get out of sync. And that disrupted circadian rhythm can affect all the functions of the body. Experts note that "circadian confusion" causes problems throughout our body. Some of the most exciting new lighting technologies for sleep problems mimic our personal circadian rhythm.

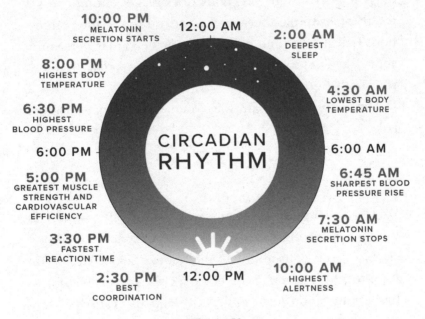

10:00 PM
MELATONIN
SECRETION STARTS

12:00 AM

2:00 AM
DEEPEST
SLEEP

8:00 PM
HIGHEST BODY
TEMPERATURE

4:30 AM
LOWEST BODY
TEMPERATURE

6:30 PM
HIGHEST
BLOOD PRESSURE

6:00 PM

CIRCADIAN
RHYTHM

6:00 AM

6:45 AM
SHARPEST BLOOD
PRESSURE RISE

5:00 PM
GREATEST MUSCLE
STRENGTH AND
CARDIOVASCULAR
EFFICIENCY

7:30 AM
MELATONIN
SECRETION STOPS

3:30 PM
FASTEST
REACTION TIME

2:30 PM
BEST
COORDINATION

12:00 PM

10:00 AM
HIGHEST
ALERTNESS

Figure 11

When you don't sleep enough, your body needs to find ways to stay alert, so it keeps pumping out chemicals to try to keep you from dozing off. Your body isn't designed to have these neurochemicals firing off all the time. As a result, you are at greater risk of high blood pressure, diabetes, depression, heart attacks, and even strokes. For example, data suggests people who sleep less than six hours per night can be four times as likely to have a heart attack.

Ways Sleep Impacts Your Cancer Risk

Some of the things I mentioned about sleep probably don't surprise you—especially the part about feeling irritable or foggy-headed when your body doesn't get enough rest. I use these examples because I want you to see the connection. The amount and quality of your sleep may determine your risk of getting some types of cancer as well as how well your body fights cancer.

There are three main ways poor sleep impacts cancer risk.

Weight Gain

We know that poor sleep can cause weight gain—which, as we have seen, increases your risk of cancer. Remember, sleep impacts your ability to metabolize sugar. When you have too little sleep, your body secretes more insulin to lower your blood sugar. A lack of sleep also causes disruption with other hormones related to weight and hunger— such as leptin and ghrelin. Basically, these tell you when you're hungry and full. Poor sleep makes these hormones go in the wrong direction and can cause overeating. There is a fascinating study recently published that shows staying up at night watching TV can cause the "munchies." As we all know, the foods we eat when we have the munchies are almost always low on nutrition and high in calories. They also can cause acid reflux, which makes it hard to have a good sleep. I guess you're not choosing hummus and carrots late at night, are you?!

Weakened Immunity

Some studies have shown that even just one night of sleeping only four or five hours can decrease the number of our natural killer cells—those critical cells that are used to fight cancer. That doesn't mean that if you miss a few hours of sleep a few nights that you are going to get cancer. But chronic sleep deprivation over many years is likely impacting your immunity.

Research also shows that if you have several sleepless nights a week, you could have fewer cytokines—those proteins that help fight infections. Surprised? Think about this. What do you do when you have the flu? You stay home and in bed—and you sleep! Why? Because your body needs that sleep to help fight the infection. So, if you have chronic sleep problems, it seems to make sense that your immunity functions might be impaired—which can put you at greater risk for cancer.

Abnormal Cell Behavior

When your circadian rhythm is "messed up," it may cause abnormal behavior in cells that can lead to the development of cancer and then unusually aggressive growth of these cells. It also causes direct damage to DNA. Some studies have shown that poor sleep speeds up aging, which leads to a normal decrease in immunity. We all know that we look older when we don't get enough sleep—but I'm talking about your cells prematurely aging! If your cells age too soon, that puts you at risk for various diseases, since important immune cells stop functioning effectively.

What's Behind the Sleep–Cancer Connection?

Several hormones and neurotransmitters including dopamine, serotonin, norepinephrine, and orexin are involved in sleep. The two, though, that may be most related to sleep and its impact on cancer that strike me as most important are cortisol and melatonin.

We'll start with cortisol. Sometimes people refer to cortisol as the stress hormone. It helps to manage stress by regulating our blood pressure, our heart rate, our mood, and even our blood sugar. Like adrenaline, it can help us prepare for battle! It also works to treat inflammation. But when cortisol gets out of control, it can disrupt the normal functioning in our body. At a certain level, cortisol can begin to damage our DNA—damage that allows cells to mutate into cancer cells and grow uncontrollably.

Cortisol's importance to sleep relates to its "diurnal variation," meaning it peaks in the morning—causing us to wake up!—and then declines throughout the day. Stress and sleep are related, when cortisol is high or low. By this I mean, when we don't get enough sleep, we are prone to stress. And when we sleep too much, it might be a component of stress. People who wake up repeatedly during the night are also more likely to have abnormal cortisol patterns. It may be a high cortisol level that's causing this awakening. Your body is tricked into thinking it is time to get up.

Cortisol also plays an important role in our immune response. Several studies have shown it causes the body to release white blood cells when there is immediate stress. It can also reduce inflammation. When stress becomes chronic and we're churning out cortisol regularly, our bodies start to become resistant, and we have the opposite effect on immune function—weakening it, instead of strengthening it. It now increases inflammation when we should be decreasing it.

I mentioned the potential consequences of working night shifts—shift work—on cancer risk. Disruption of the biological clock can wreak havoc on your body's immune response. Some studies have shown that female night shift workers have higher rates of breast cancer—30 to 60 percent higher—than women who sleep normal hours. It seems that they are more likely to have a "shifted cortisol rhythm" in which their cortisol levels peak in the afternoon. They also are fighting the effect of melatonin, which is telling them it's time to sleep. Several studies show those women who engage in shift work typically die earlier from breast cancer. Shift work may also increase the risk of other cancers, such as brain, leukemia, non-Hodgkin's lymphoma, and prostate cancer.

We've seen similar patterns with firefighters who demonstrate increased risk for cancer. Their risks include environmental toxins and stress but also disrupted sleep. Granted, there are other factors that play a role but let's stop dismissing the importance of sleep.

Melatonin

The other hormone that has a big impact on sleep and cancer risk is melatonin. This is a popular supplement some of you may have tried for sleep. Melatonin is produced by the brain during sleep. Technically, it's the suprachiasmatic nucleus—that master clock I referenced earlier—that decides how and when to release melatonin. Its main job is to regulate night and day cycles, which then drives your sleep-wake cycles. It is naturally suppressed by light and triggered by the dark. Darkness causes the body to produce more melatonin, which signals the body to prepare for sleep, and light decreases melatonin production and signals the body to prepare for being awake. Unlike cortisol, it increases in the evening and for most people peaks around 3:00 or 4:00 a.m. and then falls to lows around midmorning. It seems that some people who have trouble sleeping have low levels of melatonin. If you're up all night, you may not be producing enough melatonin.

Research shows that low levels of melatonin may increase the risk for several cancers. This likely relates to melatonin's effect on estrogen as well. Often when melatonin is low, estrogen levels are high. This might explain low melatonin sometimes seen in patients with breast, endometrial, prostate, and ovarian cancer, which have all been tied to estrogen.

What's particularly interesting about melatonin when it comes to cancer prevention is that it seems to have antioxidant properties that help prevent damage to cells. Antioxidants might sound like a bad word since it contains the word "anti." But antioxidants—like antibodies—are a good thing. They can help prevent the growth of new cancer-nurturing blood vessels as well as fight free radicals from causing damage to cells. Remember, damage to cells is what can lead to cancer, so anything that helps prevent damage might lower the risk of cancer.

Please recognize that I am not suggesting that you should start taking melatonin as part of your cancer prevention program. Rather, I want you to recognize the importance of sleep and strive to get quality sleep every night. If you have trouble sleeping, I want you to talk to your doctor about different strategies that might improve sleep, including the possible use of melatonin. Melatonin supplements are mostly made in a lab; check with your doctor, since it can interfere with medications such as blood thinners, blood pressure drugs, birth control pills, anti-seizure medications, and some immune-suppressing drugs. Some foods such as walnuts, olives, tomatoes, strawberries, cherries, and cow's milk also contain melatonin. That helps explain why a warm glass of milk before bed has been a common remedy for insomnia. Some of tryptophan is metabolized into melatonin. Your grandmother had it right!

You may be wondering if you should get a test for your cortisol or melatonin level. At this point in time, I don't advise people to get these tests. There's a big range of what is normal, and it can be hard to interpret these tests since the levels vary during the day.

How Much Sleep Do You Need?

Your sleep needs are going to be different than your spouse, child, or sibling. Everyone is a little different. But in general, most adults need about seven and a half to eight hours of sleep daily. There are people with some genetic variation who need less sleep, but they are exceptions. Age also plays a role as we get older but not as much as you think. We tend to have more trouble falling asleep and maintaining sleep as we get older, but overall sleep needs don't change much.

How do you know your ideal sleep time and the amount of sleep your body needs? There are different methods, such as sleep diaries, trackers and monitors, and sleep labs, that can help.

At the simplest level, ask yourself—if you didn't set an alarm clock, how late would you likely sleep? When you do set an alarm, do you constantly hit the snooze button? If that's the case, your body needs more sleep.

One method I often use with patients is a "sleep vacation." The name is a bit misleading since it's more of an experiment than a vacation. This is an especially good test for those of you that rely on alarms. Here's how it works. You need to pick a time over a two-week period when you don't have to wake up at a specific time, since for this "vacation" you are not going to use an alarm. During the first two to three days, you may be anxious because there's no alarm. Don't count those days. Go to bed the same time every night and allow yourself to wake up naturally. Over those two weeks, you will develop a pattern of sleeping that fits your needs. For most people, it will likely be around seven or eight hours, plus or minus an hour. I like this experiment because it helps you find out—not simply guess—how much sleep your body needs. There are some people—very few—who have a "short sleep phenotype" that allows them to function with only five hours of sleep, with no harmful effects. Don't assume, though, that you have that phenotype! The "sleep vacation" helps many people find out they aren't sleeping enough.

For those of you that are "techies" and like a lot of data, you also can use trackers on your smartwatches, tablets, and even your bed and pajamas! I do think those are helpful to look at trends over time. I have been using one over the past year and there is a good correlation between how I feel in the morning and my sleep score. Even more so, when I get a "low score" indicating poor quality sleep, I renew my efforts to get better sleep. That's what I find is the best aspect of these trackers—continuous personal feedback that demonstrates the relationship between your sleep and your health. If you keep getting low scores and feel lousy, that also clearly shows you aren't getting enough sleep.

Solving Your Sleep Problems

The push for better sleep is not an easy battle. It requires effort and a variety of strategies. In recent years, the concept of cognitive behavioral therapy for insomnia (CBT-I) has gained more acceptance in the medical community. The American College of Physicians issued a guideline in 2016 suggesting it as first-line treatment for chronic sleep problems. The focus is on changing thoughts, beliefs, attitudes, and behaviors that contribute to insomnia. CBT-I can give the proper information about age-related sleep changes, reasonable and practical sleep goals, as well as the influence of naps, food, and exercise. It's effective at teaching important sleep habits, which translates into quality sleep.

Components typically include:

Stimulus control therapy. This method helps remove factors that condition your mind to resist sleep. For example, you might be coached to use the bed only for sleep and sex. No Netflix bingeing anymore in bed! No daytime napping either with this approach. The more you stay in bed without sleeping conditions your brain to not associate the brain with sleep. So, if you can't fall asleep within twenty minutes or so, you often need to get out of bed until you are sleepy.

Sleep restriction. Sleep restriction therapy (SRT) is based on the belief that lying in bed when you are awake can become a bad habit that leads to poor sleep. It is a type of chronotherapy, which controls exposure to sleep to help create a consistent sleep schedule. We aren't actually restricting sleep but rather restricting the amount of time you lie awake in bed without sleeping. It starts with decreasing the time you spend in bed, making you sleepy during the day, which makes you more tired the next night. Once your sleep improves, your time in bed gradually increases. This may sound harsh, and it's not for everyone, but it has shown some success when done over several weeks. Usually a doctor or therapist is needed to help do this correctly, and some people with underlying health conditions such as seizures or bipolar disease should not use this technique.

Sleep compression. Sleep compression is another option that's similar to sleep restriction but less intense. It starts with distinguishing your total sleep time vs. your time in bed. If you need seven and a half hours of sleep a night but you're in bed for nine hours, you decrease the amount of time in bed by fifteen to thirty minutes a week. You gradually compress bed time over several weeks to approach your sleep needs. You are training your body to sleep when you are in bed.

Paradoxical intention. How often do you get stressed and fearful that you can't fall asleep, which just makes it worse? You can't fall asleep for hours and are getting more and more stressed about it. You essentially are experiencing performance anxiety when it comes to sleep. With this technique, you get into bed and stay awake—on purpose. When you engage your feared behavior of staying awake, performance anxiety related to trying to fall asleep slowly diminishes. It's not meant to be an episode of *Fear Factor,* but acknowledging the fear will help reduce your anxiety and enable you to sleep easier. It's not for everyone but when done correctly can help address the anxiety that you may have when it's bedtime.

Biofeedback. This method tries to help you become more aware of your body's responses, especially those that are usually involuntary such as heart rate, breathing, muscle tension, and blood pressure. It then teaches you how to adjust them. The idea behind biofeedback is that, by harnessing the power of your mind and becoming aware of what's going on inside your body, you can gain more control over how you sleep.

Progressive muscle relaxation. I know some people still "count sheep" when they have trouble falling asleep. Others count backward—I have one patient who counts backward subtracting 7 from 1,000—she complains of trouble falling asleep and I tell her to stop doing math at bedtime! Instead, we need to quiet our mind. One technique that has been getting a lot of attention in recent years—although the concept has been around for over a century—is progressive muscle relaxation. The premise is that mental calmness results from physical relaxation. You might be having trouble falling asleep because you are either physically tense or mentally active. So, we need to address both to maximize good sleep. Experts recommend tensing and relaxing muscle groups one at a time in a specific order, generally beginning with the lower extremities and ending with the face and chest.

Here is how it works: Lie in bed as if you are about to fall asleep. While breathing in, contract one muscle group (for example your upper thighs or abdominal wall) for five to ten seconds, then exhale and suddenly release the tension in that muscle group. Give yourself ten to twenty seconds to relax, and then move on to the next muscle group (for example your buttocks). While releasing the tension, try to focus on the changes you feel when the muscle group is relaxed. Gradually work your way up the body contracting and relaxing muscle groups. It takes practice but this might be what you need to help fall asleep.

For CBT-I to be most effective, it usually takes place over several weeks under the guidance of a doctor or therapist. Realistically, not everyone can find a doctor to help with this or can afford it. There are some different apps for CBT that can help you do it correctly, including a free one that is used by the US Department of Veterans Affairs called CBT-I coach. You don't have to be a veteran to use it.

Schedule Anxiety

Another option to address anxiety and stress that is affecting your sleep is to schedule it. Some experts suggest you find ten minutes a day to concentrate on the things you are worried or stressed about. (Just not at bedtime!) With daily practice, your brain can learn to compartmentalize and that becomes your "worry time," so you don't worry all throughout the day. You can get all of your worrying done at one time of the day—long before you get into bed to sleep.

Sleep Hygiene

Just as we practice good hygiene for our body, we need to practice good hygiene for our sleep. By preparing our environment and being conscious about our pre-sleep routines, we can set our bodies up for successful sleep.

Here are some of the strategies I have learned over the years to help you get some quality sleep.

Make Your Sleep Space into a Spa

By that I mean, it needs to be dark, quiet, and cool. Have you ever gone to a spa that is bright and loud? I bet not because they wouldn't be in business for very long. I will admit that spas are usually warm, but when it comes to your "sleep spa," lower the thermostat. The data shows that most people sleep better in cool temperatures. The ideal temperature? 67°F. I know that the thermostat is often a battleground in the bedroom, but cooler is better. Give it a try and see how your sleep goes.

Another tip to keep things cool—wear socks to bed. Not exactly what you suspected, is it? Wearing socks in bed increases blood flow to your feet and causes heat loss through your skin, thereby lowering your core body temperature. The role of socks and sleep is a little bit counterintuitive, but there is science to support it.

I can thank my father-in-law for this next tip: hang some room-darkening shades. I must tell you they can work wonders. There are different levels of darkening and you might lose some of the light cues for awakening if no sunlight at all can get through in the morning, but many people find success with these shades. You can even use high-quality paper ones that you tape on; they're fairly inexpensive.

For the same effect, you can just wear a sleep mask over your eyes. It keeps out the light, and many people say it helps signal and condition their brain: "enough thinking—it's time for sleep." Masks can take a couple nights getting used to, so be sure to try it more than just once or twice.

Another sensory area that you need to consider: sound. Your brain still hears and processes sound while you sleep. That's the reason the room needs to be quiet. The sounds that your brain hears can wake you up, even from deep sleep. Some of my patients use ear plugs and others use white noise machines. Personally, I just try to keep the area quiet.

One other trick to keep your sleeping area like a spa is the use of a humidifier. Some patients seem to think a humidifier is something that's in a museum, when I mention it! "Do they still sell them?" is often the retort! Using a humidifier puts moisture back in the air and can make it easier to fall and stay asleep. Humidifiers are particularly useful during the winter when the air is often dry. Dry air can cause irritation in mucosal membranes in the eyes, nose, and throat. Use distilled water if you can get it—it works best. Just be sure to clean your humidifier every day.

Keep it dark, quiet, and cool!

You Should Be Bedded for Royalty

Examine your mattress. When did you buy it? Have kids been bouncing on it? Does it sag in some places? Most experts recommend you change at least every ten years, preferably sooner. Mattresses lose their shape and firmness over time. Have you ever "sunk" into a mattress? It's not comfortable. I'm sure some of you are using the first mattress you ever bought. They can get expensive, I know, but sleeping on an old, worn-out mattress is not only bad for your back, it's bad for your sleep. My mother often complained of back pain, and, in retrospect, I think her mattress contributed to it.

What kind of mattress is best? When it comes to sleep and mattresses, you want pressure evenly distributed across your body. Firmness is a matter of personal preference. Be sure to turn the mattress 180 degrees every six months or so. That way, you don't only use one section of the mattress. Be sure to get some help when turning it. It's harder to do than it seems! A good friend of mine shared some advice more than two decades ago that's good to repeat: "John, you spend a third of your life in bed. It's the one place you spend the most time in your life—probably more than work. Make the mattress comfortable."

Examine those sheets too! I'm not talking about thread count, although 300 to 400 would be a good goal. When it comes to sheets, the key is to not forget about changing and cleaning them. Most experts suggest cleaning at least every two weeks. Don't get grossed out, but body oils, dead skin cells, and perspiration linger in your sheets. (We shed 500 million skin cells every day!) Bacteria and dust mites also accumulate. Some people suggest your sheets have more germs than a toilet seat! All of this can cause irritation to your skin and throat, worsening conditions such as asthma and eczema.

Although our moms were right to tell us to make our beds every morning, you don't have to do it right away. Moisture builds up in our sheets during sleep. It's a good idea to let the sheets breathe a little after you wake up— that way, they attract fewer bacteria.

Ever try a weighted blanket? There are a wide range of quilts and comforters on the market now that can weigh between five and thirty pounds. This extra weight seems to provide a gentle pressure that can give the feeling of being held. Some research suggests this type of pressure can cause the release of serotonin, a neurotransmitter that helps promote sleep. I have tried these blankets and do think they can help with sleep. One of my sons had some trouble sleeping and a weighted blanket seems to have done the trick in getting him to have more restful sleep.

For me, the most important part of the bed for good sleep is my pillow. The pillow for your head should support the natural curve of your neck and be comfortable. Many of us seem to have our head and neck on it too high or too low. A pillow that's too high can put your neck into a position that causes muscle strain on your back, neck, and shoulders, and one that's too low causes hyperextension. The pillow should ordinarily maintain a height of four to six inches to support the head and neck (and shoulders when lying on the back).

Some people suggest sleeping with no pillow. I am not a fan of this approach, since it can eventually cause neck pain if there is poor alignment. Basically, it comes down to personal preference. If you have trouble sleeping or wake up with neck, arm, or back pain, experiment with a different pillow as well as how high you lie on it.

One trick my wife does is to spray lavender on the pillow. Some data suggests aromatherapy increases deep sleep, perhaps by slowing heart rate and lowering blood pressure and temperature—which can help one feel more rested. It might be worth a try! You can even try an air diffuser in the bedroom.

What about pets in your bed? Good news! Allowing your pet to sleep in your bed can help with sleep. Studies show that having a dog in the bed can help relieve insomnia by lowering anxiety and modifying hyperarousal and hypervigilance. A dog's rhythmic breathing, when one lies next to you, can help lull you to sleep. Cats help too. Many cat lovers talk about how the purring sound soothes them. Pets in the bed might even increase flow of oxytocin, a "feel-good" hormone. Just remember to clean the sheets a bit more often.

Change your sheets frequently, turn the mattress every six months, reposition your pillow, and invite your pets to be cuddle buddies!

Establish a Regular Schedule

When it comes to sleep, a regular schedule is critical. Many of us are over-scheduled. We are trying to accomplish too many things with limited time. Work, family, friends—it's challenging to fit everything in during twenty-four hours.

The issue for most people is not in creating a schedule. The problem, I have found, is that we don't stick to a regular schedule—with emphasis on the word "regular." Something always seems to come up that makes you modify your schedule—and your sleeping time is what usually gets cut down. And that goes back to the fact that most of us don't realize the importance of sleep, so we are quick to sacrifice it.

If you set a goal to go to sleep at 10:00 or 11:00 p.m. and wake up at 7:00 a.m., then try to stick to it every day. Of course, there are going to be exceptions—that's just how life is. But you can't be having a different schedule every day or every few days.

Best way to adhere to a schedule? Set an alarm and stick to it. No hitting the snooze button! You should consider deleting the "snooze" function if you use an alarm app. I know many of you won't want to hear this but there is no "sleep bank." You can't work crazy hours all week and then think you can make up for it on the weekend. Sleep and its relationship to our health is all about it being consistent and regular. Yes, it would be great if we could sleep extra hours one day and sleep less the other—"put away" some hours now to use them later. Your body just doesn't work that way. You feel better on the days that you sleep longer. But you still cause damage on the days when you don't sleep enough or get quality sleep. This means that a couple of good nights of sleep don't negate the many bad nights. Consistency counts!

Check Your Medications

Medications are one of the top disruptors of sleep. Numerous medications—both prescription and over the counter—may impact your ability to get a good night's sleep, and I bet you don't even realize it. For instance, within the last few years, there has been a trend—supported by research—to take medicine for high blood pressure in the evening, rather than in the morning. Since some high blood pressure medicines have a component of a diuretic—you can end up having to get up at night to urinate, interrupting your sleep. Other medications known to impact sleep include:

- Steroids, including prednisone
- Respiratory inhaled medications
- Diet pills
- ADD and ADHD drugs
- Some antidepressants

Nonprescription drugs that can cause sleep problems include:

- Pseudoephedrine, including the brand Sudafed
- Drugs with caffeine, including the brands Anacin, Excedrin, and NoDoz, as well as some cough and cold medications
- Illegal drugs such as cocaine, amphetamines, and methamphetamines
- Nicotine, which can disrupt sleep and reduce total sleep time; smokers report more daytime sleepiness than do nonsmokers, especially in younger age groups

Don't stop any of these required medications without talking to your doctor. Sometimes sleeping issues caused by these medicines might be able to be solved through changing the dose or the time of day you take them.

As for sleeping pills, they can be a double-edged sword. Sleeping pills work best and are safest if you use them for a short time along with lifestyle changes. They are meant to be a temporary treatment. They should not be used for the rest of your life, as medicine for high blood pressure and heart disease should. They do have side effects, too, such as drowsiness during the day, constipation, headaches, changes in appetite, occasional weakness, and nausea. Worse, they can cause dependence, either physically or psychologically. They can be very hard to come off, especially since they can cause a "rebound insomnia" when you initially stop taking them, causing a difficult cycle to break. There also is some data that sleeping pills induce more non-REM sleep, and we still need to learn the right relationship between REM and non-REM sleep. Bottom line: research shows that lifestyle and behavior changes are the best long-term choices to help you sleep well.

A note about caffeine and coffee. The data that has been collected on caffeine's effect on sleep hasn't been consistent. In theory, caffeinated beverages block a brain chemical called adenosine that promotes sleep. In practice, while some studies do show coffee makes it harder to fall asleep, others say it has no effect. I'm going to be honest—I enjoy coffee, especially in the morning. I rarely drink it in the evening, but I have on occasion without difficulty. That's just me; many friends and family members can't have a cappuccino after dinner unless it's decaf (decaf coffee still has some caffeine!). I recommend you do your own test. If you have a cup after 3:00 or 4:00 p.m., and it keeps you up, then make it a point not to have caffeine past noon.

Put the Screens Away

How many of you use the time when you get into bed to catch up on your social media, or just to "go over emails." Bedtime is not the time or place for social media catch-up and to be on your screens. Remember, you want to quiet your mind when you prepare to sleep. How often does email or a social media post create an emotional response from you? That's not what you want before sleep. Almost everything we do on phones and tablets is stimulating to our brains, especially social media, texting, email, and on-line shopping.

The other problem with screens before bed is blue light. I have had patients say their screens don't emit blue light, but it's not a light color we can see with our eyes. Blue light is a wavelength emitted from many of our digital devices. It turns out some of the energy-efficient lighting we all have become enamored with also increases our exposure to blue light. The problem with blue light is that it can suppress the body's release of melatonin, making it more challenging to fall asleep, because your body thinks it's time to wake up. Some good news—the amount of blue light from newer devices seems to be less of a problem nowadays. Even if you own a newer device, it's still a bad idea to use it before bed.

What about those fancy glasses? Is it time to buy some of those blue-light blocking glasses? The American Optometric Association does not recommend spending money on blue light glasses to improve sleep. Rather, they suggest simply decreasing evening screen time and set devices to night mode.

How many of you put the phone on your nightstand? Do you put it in sleep or airplane mode? If not, make sure your phone goes to sleep when you do! No email or text will be so urgent that you need to keep it next to you—just in case. If it's really necessary, you can program your phone to allow certain numbers to ring through the sleep mode. Don't be a "JIC-er"—those folks who keep their phones nearby "just in case." I always ask people "just in case" what? There's not usually a practical answer! A friend of mine puts her phone in the closet before she goes to bed. Most of you probably aren't willing to do that—she says it takes a few days to get used to, but she swears she sleeps better and is less stressed every morning! It might be worth a try!

Don't Become an Orthosomniac

Here's a new word for you: "orthosomnia." It describes an unhealthy obsession with the amount of sleep you are getting. If you have multiple apps and trackers and are discussing your sleep patterns with friends and family, you might be too focused on your sleep. Personally, while I do think sleep trackers and apps can play an important role in evaluating your sleep, I'm not sure you need to be tracking it most days. The irony is that too much focus on tracking may make your sleep worse. You will experience anxiety if you don't like what your numbers are showing. The desire for "perfect" sleep may result in sleep habits that don't result in restorative sleep. Focus more on the goal rather than specific data points.

Summary

Sleep deprivation is a stress on your body that increases your risk of disease. Getting quality sleep is critical for your overall health as well as your personal cancer prevention strategy. Make restful sleep a priority, and when you have problems with sleep, talk to your doctor and other professionals to help make the changes you need to be well rested every day. Sleep disorders are common, but they are also treatable. Better sleep leads to better health and plays a role in decreasing your risk of cancer. Take control of your sleep and you will take control of your cancer risk.

WHAT ABOUT NAPS? Some cultures incorporate naps into their daily lives. The key is to nap smartly. That means if you take a nap sometimes, do it in the afternoon for no more than twenty minutes. Don't do it past 3:00 p.m., since napping too late will mess up your bedtime routine. You might consider drinking some coffee right before your nap; by the time the caffeine activates, you will be ready to wake up and it might help you be even more refreshed.

ANSWERS

1. **FALSE**—Sleep needs do not change much as you get older. You don't sleep as deeply as you age but the total amount of necessary sleep doesn't change much.

2. **TRUE**—Data has demonstrated that shift work can increase your risk for certain types of cancer.

3. **TRUE**—Low levels of melatonin have been linked to some cancers. This doesn't mean you should take melatonin supplements; rather, focus on quality sleep.

4. **FALSE**—You should delete the snooze button on your phone, and not use one on a clock. If you need to press snooze, that likely means you aren't getting enough sleep.

5. **FALSE**—Most people do not need to nap. Taking naps during the day may make it more difficult to sleep at night.

CHAPTER NINE

Can't I Just
Wait for a Vaccine?

TRUE OR FALSE?

1. We have a vaccine that protects against cancer.
2. A vaccine against cancer could cause you to get cancer.
3. The side effects of vaccines are not well known.
4. Vaccines inject cancer into your body so you can develop immunity.
5. The safety track record of vaccines is both good and bad.

(Answers at end of chapter)

"I DON'T LIKE THE FLU SHOT. One year, it gave me the flu," Ann retorts every fall when I recommend the flu shot. Some years, she decides to get the flu shot. Others, she doesn't. She has been getting it more often the last couple of years. Ever since she had a bad case of shingles—and wished she had taken the shingles vaccine that could have prevented it—she's become more willing to discuss the usefulness of vaccines. Ann does a lot of reading online about vaccines, but she doesn't always check the sources of her information. "I can tell what's right or not" is the typical response when I ask patients how they judge what they read. Unfortunately, there is a lot of misunderstanding and misinformation about vaccines, especially as it relates to cancer.

One day, I do expect us to find cures for most cancers and to develop therapies that are even more effective. Until then, we need to develop our personalized cancer prevention plan as we have discussed over the past eight chapters: focus on screening recommendations, restorative sleep, the food we eat, how active we are—and getting immunizations. Just as you get immunized for some diseases such as measles or pneumonia, you need to get vaccinated against some types of cancer.

How surprised are you when I say there is a vaccine for cancer? Do you believe me? Well, the truth is, vaccines do exist—but only for a few types of cancer.

Vaccines are one of the great discoveries of medicine. They help prevent us from getting certain diseases. Many of you reading this book have never experienced chickenpox, mumps, or the measles because we have vaccines. These vaccines trigger antibodies to fight infection, giving us immunity to defend against disease.

When it comes to cancer, there are two types of vaccines:

1. Prevention vaccines
2. Therapeutic vaccines

Prevention Vaccines

Prevention vaccines are the type with which you are likely most familiar. As its name implies, it prevents you from getting a disease. They key is you must get the vaccine before you get the disease; otherwise it doesn't work. Examples of prevention vaccines include measles/mumps/rubella, chickenpox, meningitis, and influenza.

Only two types of cancer prevention vaccines are approved by the FDA.

Human Papillomavirus (HPV) Vaccine

The human papillomavirus (HPV) is a common sexually transmitted disease. There are many different types of HPV, and some have been shown to cause various forms of cancer, as well as genital warts. HPV infections cause more than 32,000 cases of cancer in the United States each year, and many more worldwide. The good news is that the HPV vaccine protects against cervical, vaginal, and vulvar cancer. The bad news is that people often mistakenly believe that it is just for women, but it also protects against penile cancer in men. And for both sexes, it defends against anal cancer and genital warts. It also protects against certain head and neck cancers, including those of the tonsils and throat. The current vaccine protects against 90 percent of HPV-related cancers.

The most recent CDC recommendation is to start immunization at age eleven or twelve, although vaccination can be started as early as age nine. They also recommend vaccination for everyone through age twenty-six if not adequately vaccinated previously. HPV vaccination is given as a series of either two or three doses, depending on one's age at initial vaccination.

Vaccination is not recommended for those older than age twenty-six. However, some adults ages twenty-seven through forty-five years may decide to get the HPV vaccine after discussion with their doctor if they did not get adequately vaccinated when they were younger. It may be less effective, however, since you must be vaccinated before exposure, and people in this age range, especially those who are sexually active, may have already been exposed to HPV.

Even though this vaccine can prevent cancer related to HPV, vaccination rates have been low—some estimate 50 percent for teens. There are a couple reasons for this that you should be aware of.

First, I think there is confusion about which virus we're vaccinating against. I still have parents say to me, "There's a vaccine for HIV?" even though this is HPV—two completely different diseases. Second, there seems to be a mistaken belief that getting the HPV vaccine will encourage adolescents to be more sexually promiscuous. There is no evidence that giving the HPV vaccine is linked with higher sexual activity. In fact, a recent article reviewing studies of more than 500,000 individuals revealed that there was no increase in sexual activity after HPV vaccination.

Hepatitis B

The other preventive vaccine is for hepatitis B. You may be thinking that hepatitis B is not a type of cancer. You're right. Hepatitis B is an infection of the liver. Chronic infection with hepatitis B, however, can cause liver cancer. If we prevent you from getting hepatitis B, we likely will reduce your risk from getting liver cancer. Hepatitis C also causes liver cancer, but we currently only have treatment for hepatitis C, not a vaccine. Keep in mind that liver cancer has low survival rates, with less than 20 percent of people alive five years after diagnosis. Preventing liver cancer is a good idea, and vaccination is an effective strategy.

I bet you didn't know that the hepatitis B vaccine was the first anti-cancer vaccine ever created. Even though it's been around since the mid-1980s, it wasn't recommended for routine vaccination of infants until 1991!

The hepatitis B vaccine is usually given as two, three, or four shots. The CDC recommends that infants get their first dose of hepatitis B vaccine at birth and usually complete the series at six months of age. Children and adolescents younger than nineteen years of age who have not yet gotten the vaccine should also be vaccinated.

Because the vaccine wasn't given to many of you reading this book, you might want to consider getting vaccinated.

The CDC also recommends the hepatitis B vaccine for certain unvaccinated adults:

- People whose sex partners have hepatitis B
- Sexually active persons who are not in a long-term monogamous relationship
- People seeking evaluation or treatment for a sexually transmitted disease
- Men who have sexual contact with other men
- People who share needles, syringes, or other drug-injection equipment
- People who have household contact with someone infected with the hepatitis B virus

- Health care and public safety workers at risk for exposure to blood or body fluids
- Residents and staff of facilities for developmentally disabled persons
- People in correctional facilities
- Victims of sexual assault or abuse
- Travelers to regions with increased rates of hepatitis B
- People with chronic liver disease, kidney disease, HIV infection, infection with hepatitis C, or diabetes
- Anyone who wants to be protected from hepatitis B

You may have noticed that these vaccines are preventing infections that may lead to cancer rather than directly preventing cancer itself. When it comes to cancer, we need to look at every strategy. If we know certain infections increase risk for cancer, let's do all we can to prevent those infections, which will help you to take control of your cancer risk.

I do want you to know these vaccines are safe. Vaccines undergo a rigorous testing and approval process before they are released to the public. Side effects such as fever, headache, and soreness of the injection site can occur but are usually minor. The presence of side effects does not mean that a vaccine is not safe. Vaccines have a proven track record of safety, and the benefits far outweigh any risks.

There are several other vaccines in development. For example, scientists are also working on a vaccine for colon cancer, but right now it's only for people with an inherited condition, called Lynch syndrome, which dramatically increases their risk of cancer. Lynch syndrome affects more than a million people, although less than 10 percent of those affected know they have it. The vaccine, still undergoing studies, prevents the growth of cancer cells in the colon. Given that this type of colon cancer is related to a genetic mutation, it's not certain it will work in a broader population. As more people do genetic testing and learn about hereditary cancer syndromes, these types of vaccines likely will become more important in saving lives.

Therapeutic Vaccines

The other type of vaccinations for cancer are therapeutic vaccines. These are not the type of vaccines that we typically think of since they are designed to help treat cancer when you already have it, rather than prevent it. They are a type of immunotherapy, so it can be confusing that they are called vaccines.

We consider them vaccines because they help to boost the body's natural defenses to fight a cancer. It's really quite fascinating. Researchers identify targets on a patient's tumors that can help distinguish cancer cells from normal cells. Targeting the bad cells may slow or even stop a tumor from growing. In some cases, it might even destroy any cancer cells in the body after other treatments have been used. Their effectiveness is limited, and they usually work best for smaller tumors or those that are in early stages.

Currently, the FDA has approved three therapeutic vaccines.

Provenge (Sipuleucel-T)

This is a vaccine approved for men with metastatic prostate cancer that is no longer responding to hormone therapy. As a result, it's not currently used at the beginning of treatment. Provenge stimulates a patient's own immune system against cancer. What's really fascinating is that each patient has a vaccine made specifically for them using their own white blood cells. It's truly personalized. These cells are removed through a special procedure, then exposed to a protein from prostate cancer cells and a stimulatory molecule. This gets the white blood cells ready to attack the cancer cells when they are re-injected into the body. It's usually done three separate times. This isn't a cure for prostate cancer, but it may help some men live longer. I do think we will continue to see improvements in this type of vaccine over the next few years.

Bacillus Calmette-Guerin (BCG)

This is a vaccine that was originally developed to prevent tuberculosis (TB) and is now also used to treat bladder cancer. If you live in the United States, you probably haven't heard of it. That's because tuberculosis is not common here. In addition, the vaccine interferes with the test commonly used to screen for TB. However, in other areas of the world where TB is common, the BCG vaccine is often given to infants and children.

BCG plays a significant role in treating early-stage bladder cancer. Unlike most vaccines, it's not a shot in the arm. Rather, it's inserted directly into the bladder tumor. For certain types of bladder cancer, it can be up to 70 percent effective, helping to keep the cancer from growing and keep it from coming back.

Talimogene laherparepvec T-VEC (Imlygic)

This vaccine is used in patients with melanoma whose cancer cannot be removed completely with surgery or if it comes back after surgery. It's injected directly into the cancer, roughly every two weeks for several months. It then multiplies in the cancer cells and attacks them. Imlygic is a modified herpes virus, which shows the ingenuity required to fight cancer!

Like the preventive vaccines, these therapeutic vaccines are also safe. Side effects can include chills, fever, back pain, and headaches. In addition, since therapeutic vaccines target certain proteins on abnormal cells, if normal cells also express the same protein, there can be a misdirected immune response, leading to more side effects. That's why these vaccines are only given if you have cancer.

Why Don't We Have More Progress?

If you think about all the advances we have made in medicine, you might wonder why we don't have more vaccines for cancer.

There are a couple of reasons it is taking so long to discover preventive vaccines. Part of the reason is vaccines are typically designed to fight infections that might invade your body. Cancer cells often resemble normal cells, so sometimes it can be hard to distinguish the normal cells from the abnormal cells. Cancer cells also engage in similar functions as our normal cells, but they do it in a way that is abnormal and unusually fast. We don't want to kill normal cells as well as abnormal cells, since that causes a bunch of problems. It's a real challenge.

I am happy to report that numerous trials are underway for vaccines in a variety of cancers, including brain, breast, cervical, colorectal, lung, and kidney. The bad news is that we need to develop a more sophisticated approach to discovering these vaccines and making sure they are safe and effective. The discovery process often takes decades, with lots of false starts.

Artificial intelligence is playing a key role in accelerating vaccine development. This technology allows us to look at patterns more quickly and comprehensively than we can by ourselves. The processing power is immense, much faster than the human brain. Researchers in Australia announced in 2019 that they developed a flu vaccine solely through artificial intelligence. I don't think we are quite there for cancer vaccines, but it demonstrates a bright future. I'm optimistic!

We also need to recognize that we use the word "cancer" as one word, but cancer is not a single disease. It's a group of diseases that consist of abnormal cells with uncontrolled growth. Even within a certain body part, such as the breast or colon, cancers vary greatly in how they behave. Because of that, I'm doubtful we will have a vaccine for all types of cancer as a single shot, as we do for some other diseases. But I can live with that. As long as we can prevent cancer, I really don't care how many shots we need. Do you?

Summary

Vaccines play an important role in your overall health—and they also play a critical role in helping prevent cancer. As you begin to take control of your cancer risk, you need to include a personalized vaccination plan. Most people do not realize that certain infections can increase your risk of developing cancer, so make sure you are up-to-date on your vaccinations. Vaccine development is an exciting area that will continue to see advances, especially since the expedited work on coronavirus. Check with your doctor and see if you are due for any cancer prevention vaccines. You're not only protecting yourself from viral diseases, you are also helping to guard yourself against cancer.

ANSWERS

1. **FALSE**—Although we have a couple of targeted vaccines to prevent cancer, no vaccine prevents most cancers.

2. **FALSE**—A vaccine against cancer does not cause you to develop cancer.

3. **FALSE**—The side effects of vaccines are well known, and usually consist of soreness, headache, and fever.

4. **FALSE**—Vaccines do not inject cancer into your body. Typically, they contain a protein that helps the body develop an immune response.

5. **FALSE**—The safety track record of vaccines is good. It is not mixed. There is a national tracking system—Vaccines Adverse Event Reporting System—that closely monitors vaccines and alerts health care professionals, regulators, and the public about any problems.

CONCLUSION

Pulling It All Together

CONGRATULATIONS! After reading the preceding nine chapters, you now know how to reduce your odds of getting cancer. Knowledge is power and you have the power to help take control of your cancer risk. Of course, you can't eliminate your risk completely, but you can do a lot more than you might have realized. You can't change your genetics—which has little role overall in determining whether you get cancer—but you can change your lifestyle. We now know that how we live plays a big role in how long we live. The best part is you can take control of your cancer risk starting today!

- Compile a detailed family history and update it every year.
- Consider getting a genetic test, keeping in perspective what it can and cannot tell you.
- Get informed about screening guidelines. Early detection is a matter of life and death.

- Change what you eat, focusing more on a plant-based diet that emphasizes fruits and vegetables, whole grains, low-fat dairy, and fish.
- Get moving in a way that requires some exertion and gets your heart rate up most days of the week.
- Focus on restorative sleep. We've dismissed the importance of sleep for too long. It's about quantity and quality.
- Recognize a healthy mind equals a healthy body. Stop ignoring your emotions.
- Get vaccinated. Vaccines are no longer just for kids, so make sure you are up-to-date.

I also encourage you to check the sources of information when you go online to learn about cancer. Be sure to identify who wrote it and check out their credentials. Ascertain whether they have any financial interest in the information they are providing. Given how quickly advice can change in medicine, I always look at the date of content. Credible websites typically list the date the information was created.

I remain excited about the advances we are seeing in diagnostic tests and treatments for cancer, but even with this innovation, prevention remains key. It may not always seem "new" or "leading edge," or even glitzy . . . *but* . . . research consistently shows prevention works. By incorporating a cancer prevention program that is personalized for you and is part of your lifestyle, you will take control of your risk for cancer and also maximize your overall health.

ACKNOWLEDGMENTS

WRITING A BOOK CAN BE a monumental undertaking. Although my name is on the book, there are many people to recognize for making this happen.

The team at William Morris Endeavor, particularly Mel Berger, quickly embraced the concept of this book, making an idea into reality—in record time! During a global pandemic!

The amazing folks at Harper Horizon—Andrea Fleck-Nisbet, Amanda Bauch, and John Andrade—recognized the need for this book to help people prevent a leading cause of death—cancer—in this country and around the world. They have a style and a grace that makes them such a delight to work with. From day one, I felt like I was working with friends—and indeed, they are now good friends with whom I look forward to collaborating for many years.

I want to thank my WebMD colleagues, especially Kristy Hammam, Steve Peraino, Leah Gentry, Annic Jobin, Patricia Garrison, Beth Buehler, and Bob Brisco, for their willingness—and encouragement—to launch content in a book format. Consumers need to access information in different ways—and books are still one of those important strategies.

I appreciate the medical editing of my physician colleagues Dr. Michael Smith, Dr. Hansa Bhargava, Dr. Brunilda Nazario, and Dr. Neha Pathak, who helped me to explain facts and concepts in ways that people can understand. Checking facts too! Dr. John Deeken from Inova Schar Cancer Institute and Dr. Cedric Bryant from American Council on Exercise, as well as Dr. Christopher Mohr and Judah Kelly, provided guidance on various topics for which I'm most appreciative.

Kudos to Seth Wise, an illustrator and graphic artist, who I've worked with over a decade. He always brings my content to life with images that help explain what I'm trying to communicate.

I owe enormous gratitude to my friend and coworker, Kimberly Richardson, who has reviewed and edited countless versions of this book. She always encourages me to be creative in my writing style, and she helps provide me the tools to get there. She is the consummate professional.

My sisters, Charlene and Jackie, pushed me to write relatable content by making sure I didn't use too much medical jargon while at the same time always encouraging me to provide practical tips. If you seek unvarnished advice, ask family members! They always want the best for me and I have appreciated their support and encouragement throughout my life. You might have guessed—I'm the younger brother.

Thank you to my wife, Alisa, who is always a good sounding board for ideas. After hours of writing, it's important to have someone to share a good laugh with.

I want to acknowledge my sons, Luke and Jack. They are too young to have helped me write this book, but their existence made me want to write it. I want to show them that if you put your mind to something—like writing a book—you can do it. It's what my parents, John and Annamarie, always did for me. They made me feel like I could accomplish anything, and I am eternally grateful. "Johnny, you can do it" was a common refrain and no doubt gave me the skills and confidence to become a doctor and an author.

Finally, I want to thank the many patients I have worked with over the last two decades for allowing me to be part of their health care journey. There have been many laughs as well as some tears but I always strived to work together as a team. You have taught me as much as I have taught you.

Sample
One-Week Diet Plan

IN THIS PLAN, YOU WILL see several foods that you may have never tried or haven't eaten in a long time. I encourage you to keep an open mind, and give your taste buds a chance to enjoy what might be some new options for you. Remember, food is medicine!

Shopping List

Produce

- ❑ 1 pint blueberries
- ❑ 1 container blackberries
- ❑ 1 container raspberries
- ❑ 6 bananas
- ❑ Large container spinach (~16 oz.)
- ❑ 1 container arugula
- ❑ Tomatoes (7 medium)
- ❑ 1 head cauliflower
- ❑ Large bag carrots, whole
- ❑ 1 head broccoli
- ❑ Small bunch grapes

- ❑ 1 carton sliced mushrooms
- ❑ 2 large sweet potatoes
- ❑ Asparagus, 2 bunches
- ❑ 2 apples
- ❑ 1 carton blackberries
- ❑ 2 avocados
- ❑ 4 red peppers
- ❑ 1 yellow or orange pepper
- ❑ 4 small red onions
- ❑ 2 medium zucchinis
- ❑ 2 cucumbers
- ❑ 2 yellow onions
- ❑ 2 mangoes
- ❑ 3 lemons
- ❑ Bag fresh kale
- ❑ 1 carton strawberries (freeze half of carton)
- ❑ 1 individual hummus

Pantry

- ❑ 1 jar almond butter
- ❑ 1 jar peanut butter
- ❑ Honey
- ❑ Dried oats
- ❑ Walnuts
- ❑ Almonds
- ❑ Pistachios
- ❑ Dried blueberries
- ❑ Dried cherries

- ❑ Balsamic or red wine vinegar
- ❑ Extra virgin olive oil
- ❑ Italian dressing
- ❑ Coconut oil
- ❑ 2 wild-caught tuna or salmon pouches
- ❑ 3 cans low sodium black beans
- ❑ 1 can chickpeas
- ❑ 1 can salsa
- ❑ 1 can low sodium pinto beans
- ❑ 1 small jar grain mustard
- ❑ 1 small jar Kalamata olives
- ❑ Pesto sauce

Protein

- ❑ 1 dozen eggs
- ❑ 6-ounce salmon filet
- ❑ 5 large fresh raw shrimp
- ❑ Rotisserie chicken

Dairy

- ❑ Large (32-ounce) plain low-fat Greek yogurt

- ❑ Unsweetened almond milk
- ❑ Low-fat milk
- ❑ Feta cheese
- ❑ Fresh mozzarella

Frozen

- ❑ Shelled edamame
- ❑ Frozen corn
- ❑ Black bean burgers
- ❑ Premade cauliflower crust

Whole Grains

- ❑ Bag ground flaxseed
- ❑ Whole grain bread
- ❑ English muffins, whole grain
- ❑ Rice, instant brown
- ❑ Quinoa
- ❑ Soft tortilla shells, whole grain
- ❑ Dried roasted edamame
- ❑ Whole grain pasta

Miscellaneous

- ❑ Salt
- ❑ Pepper
- ❑ Garlic powder
- ❑ Dried parsley
- ❑ Red pepper flakes
- ❑ 8-ounce jar minced garlic
- ❑ Fresh basil leaves
- ❑ Paprika
- ❑ Cumin
- ❑ Fresh cilantro
- ❑ Dried oregano
- ❑ Cinnamon
- ❑ Maple syrup

Menus

An asterisk indicates an item that has a recipe in Appendix B.

Monday

BREAKFAST

- 1 cup cooked oatmeal made with dried oats and unsweetened almond milk or low-fat dairy. Top with ½ cup blueberries, ½ ounce walnuts, 1 teaspoon ground flaxseed.

LUNCH

Chicken and veggie wrap

- Spread ¼ avocado on whole grain tortilla shell. Layer rotisserie chicken, sliced red peppers, sliced zucchini, and salad greens down center of tortilla. Roll up tortilla.

SNACK

- 1 to 2 cups raw veggies (cauliflower, broccoli, and carrots) with 2 tablespoons hummus
- ½ cup fresh blackberries or raspberries

DINNER

Salmon and asparagus

- Place 1 cup asparagus and 6 ounces fish in pan with 2 tablespoons olive oil. Season with salt,

pepper, garlic powder. Bake, uncovered, at 425°
for 15 to 20 minutes or until fish flakes easily with
a fork.
- Serve with ½ cup cooked instant brown rice.

Tuesday

BREAKFAST

- 1 cup plain Greek yogurt, topped with
    ½ oz. almonds
    ½ cup blueberries
    1 teaspoon ground flaxseed

LUNCH

Edamame salad
- Mix 1 cup frozen edamame (thawed), 1 chopped
  red pepper, ½ small red onion, 1 chopped tomato,
  ¼ avocado, ¼ cup feta cheese, ¼ cup frozen corn
  (thawed), 2 tablespoons oil and vinegar
  vinaigrette.*

SNACK

- 1 no-bake energy bar*
- 1 banana and ½ cup grapes

DINNER

Loaded baked sweet potato
- Preheat oven to 425° F. Wash potato and poke holes.
  Wrap in tin foil and bake for 45 to 50 minutes.

- Top with ½ cup black beans, rinsed and drained, ½ cup diced fresh tomato, fresh cilantro, pinch of cumin, and 2 tablespoons plain Greek yogurt.

Wednesday

BREAKFAST

Egg scramble
- Cook ½ cup spinach and mushrooms, add 2 eggs, ¼ cup low sodium black beans (drained and rinsed), salt and pepper to taste.
- 1 slice whole grain toast
- ½ cup blackberries or raspberries (or your choice of seasonal fresh fruit)

LUNCH

- Pesto chicken pasta salad*

SNACK

Healthy trail mix
- 2 tablespoons dried cherries
- 2 tablespoons almonds
- 2 tablespoons walnuts
- 2 tablespoons dried blueberries

DINNER

Quick quinoa and veggies
- Make ¾ cup dried quinoa according to directions.

- While cooking, sauté 1 zucchini, ¼ cup mushrooms, 1 yellow onion, 1 red pepper with 2 tablespoons olive oil. Season with salt, pepper, and garlic powder. Mix with quinoa.

Thursday

BREAKFAST

Cherry smoothie
- 1 cup plain Greek yogurt
- ¼ cup dried cherries
- 1 banana
- 1 cup unsweetened almond milk
- Blend all ingredients. Add liquid to reach desired consistency.

LUNCH

Simple salad
- 3 cups spinach
- 1 ounce fresh mozzarella
- 2 tablespoons dried cherries
- ½ cup chopped tomatoes
- 2 tablespoons oil and vinegar vinaigrette*
- Top with 2 tablespoons walnuts and 1 wild-caught tuna or salmon pouch.

SNACK

Snack box
- 1 oz pistachios

- 1 cup raw veggies (carrots, broccoli, or peppers)
- 1 hard-boiled egg

DINNER

Easy bean tacos*
- 2 tacos (¼ cup pinto beans in each taco)
- Toppings: spinach, tomato, red onion, black beans, salsa, plain Greek yogurt

Friday

BREAKFAST

- Breakfast egg sandwich*
- 1 cup blueberries

LUNCH

- Mediterranean chickpea salad*

SNACK

- 2 sliced apples with 1 to 2 tablespoons peanut butter. Top with dried cherries, blueberries, and crushed almonds.

DINNER

Margherita pizza*
- 2 medium slices or 3 small slices

- 1 cup spinach salad with ½ cup chopped veggies (tomato, cucumber, and red pepper) and 2 tablespoons oil and vinegar vinaigrette*

Saturday

BREAKFAST

- Banana bread baked oatmeal*
- 1 cup almond milk

LUNCH

Fruit roll-up
- Spread 1 tablespoon almond butter on whole grain tortilla shell. Add sliced strawberries, banana, 1 teaspoon flax seed. Roll up.

SNACK

Smoothie
- Blend ½ cup ice, 6 ounces plain Greek yogurt, ½ banana, ½ mango, ½ cup frozen strawberries, and ¼ avocado. Add liquid (water) to reach desired consistency.

DINNER

- 1 black bean burger (cook according to package)
- Cut whole grain bread into circles for bun.
- 1 cup simple sweet potato fries*
- Top with sliced tomato, spinach, sliced onion.

Sunday

BREAKFAST

Open-faced PB&J

- Toast 2 slices whole grain bread, add 1 tablespoon peanut butter to each slice. Top with ½ cup blackberries or raspberries (or your choice of seasonal fresh fruit).
- 1 cup low-fat milk

LUNCH

Kale and veggie salad

- 2 cups fresh kale topped with ½ cup dried edamame, ½ cup cooked quinoa, ½ cup chopped veggies (tomato, cucumber, and red pepper), and 2 tablespoons oil and vinegar vinaigrette*

SNACK

Mixed fruit

- Mix ¼ sliced banana, ¼ cup blackberries, 1 chopped fresh mango, and 1 kiwi. Squeeze one fresh lemon on top.
- With 1 cup low-fat milk

DINNER

- 10-minute Mediterranean shrimp*

Sample Recipes

NO-BAKE ENERGY BARS

1 cup almond butter
1 cup dried oats
½ cup almonds (ground
   in a blender or food
   processor)

½ cup ground flaxseed
¼ cup dried blueberries
¾ cup honey

- Mix all ingredients and place on baking sheet with parchment paper.
- Refrigerate and cut into bars.

Makes approx. 10 bars
Can freeze, covered, for up to 2 months.

BREAKFAST EGG SANDWICH

1 whole grain
   English muffin

Handful spinach
1 tomato slice

1 ounce mozzarella
cheese

1 whole egg
2 egg whites

- Scramble egg in nonstick pan over medium
  high heat.
- Place cheese on one part of English muffin and
  top with scrambled egg, spinach, and tomato.
  Top with muffin and serve.

EASY BEAN TACOS

1 can pinto beans,
rinsed and drained
1 jar salsa, your choice
of spice

Soft tortilla shells,
whole grain
Desired toppings

- Warm tortilla shells in the oven on 300°F for 5 to
  10 minutes.
- Serve with spinach, tomato, red onion, pinto beans
  (rinsed and drained), salsa, and plain Greek yogurt.

MARGHERITA PIZZA

1 premade cauliflower
crust
3 pieces fresh
mozzarella cheese
sliced to ⅓ to ½ inch
thickness
1 tomato, sliced thin
5 to 6 fresh basil leaves

2 teaspoons
minced garlic
1 ½ tablespoons
olive oil
1 ½ tablespoons
balsamic vinegar
Salt and pepper
to taste

- Preheat oven to 350°F. Mix garlic and oil. Brush the cauliflower crust with oil and garlic, using half the mixture. Place in oven for 5 minutes to crisp up.
- Remove from oven and place 3 slices of cheese on top of the crust, sprinkle with salt and pepper, then place thinly sliced tomatoes on top and repeat with a sprinkling of salt and pepper.
- Place back in the oven for another 5 minutes. Watch the crust closely; if it's too dark before 2 to 3 minutes, remove it from the oven immediately.
- Meanwhile, mix the remaining oil and garlic with the balsamic vinegar, stirring until a smooth emulsion forms. Chop the basil leaves.
- Once the crust is baked and the edges are golden in color, remove from the oven, drizzle with however much of the balsamic vinegar mixture you would like, sprinkle with basil leaves, slice, and serve and enjoy!

OIL AND VINEGAR VINAIGRETTE

¾ to 1 cup extra virgin olive oil

¼ cup flax oil (optional)

½ cup balsamic vinegar (or other vinegar of your choice)

1 tablespoon Dijon mustard (or other mustard of your choice)

1 to 2 teaspoons minced garlic

½ teaspoon sea salt

- Mix all together. Store in airtight container for up to a week.

MEDITERRANEAN CHICKPEA SALAD

For the salad
1 (15-ounce) can
  chickpeas, drained
  and rinsed
1 chopped medium
  cucumber
1 chopped bell pepper
½ thinly sliced red onion
¼ cup crumbled feta
Kosher salt
Freshly ground black
  pepper

*For the lemon parsley
  vinaigrette*
¼ cup extra-virgin olive oil
⅛ cup white wine vinegar
1 tablespoon lemon juice
1 tablespoon freshly
  chopped parsley
¼ teaspoon red pepper
  flakes
Kosher salt
Freshly ground black
  pepper

- *Make salad:* In a large bowl, toss together chickpeas, cucumber, bell pepper, red onion, and feta. Season with salt and pepper.
- *Make vinaigrette:* In a jar fitted with a lid, combine olive oil, vinegar, lemon juice, parsley, and red pepper flakes. Close the jar and shake until emulsified, then season with salt and pepper.
- Dress salad with vinaigrette just before serving.

10-MINUTE MEDITERRANEAN SHRIMP

5 large shrimp, peeled
1 bunch fresh asparagus
3 tablespoons olive oil,
  divided
2 teaspoons minced
  garlic

1 whole red onion, sliced
2 teaspoons oregano
2 teaspoons paprika
1 pinch sea salt and
  ground black pepper,
  to taste

1 whole lemon, juiced

¼ cup Kalamata olives

¼ cup feta cheese

⅓ cup fresh cilantro
or parsley

- Preheat oven to 450°F.
- In a large bowl, season the shrimp with 2 tablespoons olive oil, garlic, salt, black pepper, paprika, oregano, and juice from lemon.
- Trim and wash the asparagus, then lay them flat on the baking sheet. Season with ½ tablespoon olive oil. Place seasoned shrimp on top of asparagus and top with sliced red onions.
- Bake for 10 minutes in the middle rack. Shrimp is cooked when the edges start to turn golden brown.
- Remove shrimp from oven and top with feta, olives, and fresh cilantro or parsley, drizzle with remaining olive oil and serve.

SIMPLE SWEET POTATO FRIES

1 large sweet potato, peeled

1 tablespoon olive oil

1 teaspoon garlic powder

1 teaspoon paprika

¼ teaspoon salt

½ teaspoon black pepper

- Preheat the oven to 400°F.
- Cut the sweet potatoes into sticks ¼ to ½ inch wide and 3 inches long, and toss them with the oil.
- Mix the spices, salt, and pepper in a small bowl, and toss them with the sweet potatoes. Spread them out on 2 rimmed baking sheets.

- Bake until brown and crisp on the bottom, about 15 minutes, then flip and cook until the other side is crisp, about 10 minutes. Serve hot.

BANANA BREAD BAKED OATMEAL

2 cups rolled oats
½ cup oat flour
1 teaspoon cinnamon
2 eggs
2 tablespoons ground
  flaxseed

3 mashed very ripe
  bananas (reserve ⅓
  of one for topping)
1 cup almond milk
¼ cup maple syrup
½ cup crushed walnuts
Coconut oil, for greasing

- Preheat oven to 350°F. Spray or grease an 8- to 9-inch baking dish with coconut oil.
- In a large bowl combine oats, oat flour, flaxseed, and cinnamon. Add in bananas, milk, and maple syrup and stir to combine.
- Stir in eggs before adding crushed walnuts.
- Mixture should be thick but if too thick add a bit more milk.
- Spread out in baking dish and bake for 40 minutes.
- Top with nut butter, maple syrup, or toppings of choice. Store in refrigerator and heat in microwave if left over.

PESTO CHICKEN PASTA SALAD

1 cup dry whole grain
  pasta
2 to 3 tablespoons
  prepared Italian
  salad dressing
2 tablespoons basil
  pesto sauce
1 cup fresh arugula

4 ounces shredded
  chicken (rotisserie
  chicken works well)
½ cup chopped tomatoes
1 ounce fresh
  mozzarella, cut into
  small pieces
Cracked black pepper,
  for topping

- Boil pasta for 8 to 9 minutes until tender, rinse
  with cold water, drain, and place in a large bowl.
- Add arugula, shredded chicken, tomatoes, and
  mozzarella cheese.
- Whisk together Italian salad dressing and pesto
  sauce until smooth, then pour over pasta. Toss to
  combine. Top with cracked black pepper.
- Serve immediately or cover and chill up to 8 hours
  and toss just before serving.

BLACK BEAN BURGERS

*(optional, if you prefer
  over frozen)*
1 (16-ounce) can black
  beans, drained and
  rinsed
½ green bell pepper, cut
  into 2-inch pieces
½ onion, cut into wedges

3 cloves peeled garlic
1 egg
1 tablespoon chili
  powder
1 tablespoon cumin
1 teaspoon Thai chili
  sauce or hot sauce
½ cup bread crumbs

- If grilling, preheat an outdoor grill for high heat, and lightly oil a sheet of aluminum foil. If baking, preheat oven to 375°F, and lightly oil a baking sheet.
- In a medium bowl, mash black beans with a fork until thick and pasty.
- In a food processor, finely chop bell pepper, onion, and garlic. Then stir into mashed beans.
- In a small bowl, stir together egg, chili powder, cumin, and chili sauce.
- Stir the egg mixture into the mashed beans. Mix in bread crumbs until the mixture is sticky and holds together. Divide mixture into four patties.
- If grilling, place patties on foil, and grill about 8 minutes on each side. If baking, place patties on baking sheet, and bake about 10 minutes on each side, until done.

Sample
One-Week Exercise Plan

Five-day-a-week full-body workout

Sunday

Workout Time

Moderate: 30 minutes to 45 minutes

Vigorous: 15 minutes to 20 minutes

	MODERATE	**MODERATE**	**VIGOROUS**	**VIGOROUS**
WARM UP	SETS/REPS	REST	SETS/REPS	REST
Squat stretch	3 X 10	30 seconds	2 X 15	30 seconds
EXERCISE	SETS/REPS	REST	SETS/REPS	REST
Dumbbell goblet squat	4 X 10	1 minute 30 seconds	2 X 20	45 seconds
Mountain climber jumps	4 X 15	1 minute 30 seconds	2 X 30	45 seconds
Dumbbell lunges	4 X 10 each leg	1 minute 30 seconds	2 X 15 each leg	45 seconds

Jump rope	4 X 30 seconds	1 minute 30 seconds	2 X 1 min	45 seconds
Push-up with shoulder tap	4 X 5 each arm	1 minute 30 seconds	2 X 12 each arm	45 seconds
Leg raise	4 X 10	1 minute 30 seconds	2 X 20	45 seconds

Tuesday

Workout Time

Moderate: 30 minutes to 45 minutes

Vigorous: 15 minutes to 20 minutes

	MODERATE	MODERATE	VIGOROUS	VIGOROUS
WARM UP	SETS/REPS	REST	SETS/REPS	REST
Squat stretch	3 X 10	30 seconds	2 X 15	30 seconds
EXERCISE	SETS/REPS	REST	SETS/REPS	REST
Dumbbell squat press	4 X 10	1 minute 30 seconds	2 X 20	45 seconds
Jumping jacks	4 X 30 seconds	1 minute 30 seconds	2 X 1 min	45 seconds
Dumbbell step up	4 X 10 each leg	1 minute 30 seconds	2 X 15 each leg	45 seconds
Mountain climber	4 X 30 seconds	1 minute 30 seconds	2 X 1 min	45 seconds
Side plank	4 X 30 seconds each side	1 minute 30 seconds	2 X 1 min each side	45 seconds
Leg raise	4 X 10	1 minute 30 seconds	2 X 20	45 seconds

Wednesday

Workout Time

Moderate: 30 minutes to 45 minutes

Vigorous: 15 minutes to 20 minutes

	MODERATE	MODERATE	VIGOROUS	VIGOROUS
WARM UP	SETS/REPS	REST	SETS/REPS	REST
Squat stretch	3 X 10	30 seconds	2 X 15	30 seconds
EXERCISE	SETS/REPS	REST	SETS/REPS	REST
Dumbbell shoulder press	4 X 10	1 minute 30 seconds	2 X 20	45 seconds
Dumbbell reverse lunge	4 X 8 each leg	1 minute 30 seconds	2 X 12 each leg	45 seconds
Push-up	4 X 10	1 minute 30 seconds	2 X 15	45 seconds
Jump squat	4 X 8	1 minute 30 seconds	2 X 15	45 seconds
Jump rope	4 X 30 seconds	1 minute 30 seconds	2 X 1 min	45 seconds
Leg raise	4 X 10	1 minute 30 seconds	2 X 20	45 seconds

Friday

Workout Time

Moderate: 30 minutes to 45 minutes

Vigorous: 15 minutes to 20 minutes

	MODERATE	**MODERATE**	**VIGOROUS**	**VIGOROUS**
WARM UP	SETS/REPS	REST	SETS/REPS	REST
Squat stretch	3 X 10	30 seconds	2 X 15	30 seconds
EXERCISE	SETS/REPS	REST	SETS/REPS	REST
Dumbbell goblet squat	4 X 10	1 minute 30 seconds	2 X 20	45 seconds
Dumbbell row	4 X 15	1 minute 30 seconds	2 X 30	45 seconds
Dumbbell lunges	4 X 10 each leg	1 minute 30 seconds	2 X 15 each leg	45 seconds
Mountain climber jumps	4 X 30 seconds	1 minute 30 seconds	2 X 1 minutes	45 seconds
Push-up with shoulder tap	4 X 5 each arm	1 minute 30 seconds	2 X 12 each arm	45 seconds
Jump rope	4 X 30 seconds	1 minute 30 seconds	2 X 1 minutes	45 seconds
Leg raise	4 X 10	1 minute 30 seconds	2 X 20	45 seconds

Saturday

Morning Workout Time

Moderate: 15 minutes to 20 minutes

Vigorous: 10 minutes to 15 minutes

	MODERATE	MODERATE	VIGOROUS	VIGOROUS
WARM UP	SETS/REPS	REST	SETS/REPS	REST
Squat stretch	3 X 10	30 sec	2 X 15	30 seconds
EXERCISE	SETS/REPS	REST	SETS/REPS	REST
Jump rope	4 X 30 seconds	1 minute 30 seconds	2 X 1 minutes	45 seconds
Mountain climbers	4 X 30 seconds	1 minute 30 seconds	2 X 1 minutes	45 seconds
Jumping jacks	4 X 30 seconds	1 minute 30 seconds	2 X 1 minutes	45 seconds
Leg raises	4 X 30 seconds	1 minute 30 seconds	2 X 1 minutes	45 seconds

Evening Workout Time

Moderate: 15 minutes to 20 minutes

Vigorous: 12 minutes to 15 minutes

	MODERATE	MODERATE	VIGOROUS	VIGOROUS
WARM UP	SETS/REPS	REST	SETS/REPS	REST
Squat stretch	3 X 10	30 seconds	2 X 15	30 seconds

EXERCISE	SETS/REPS	REST	SETS/REPS	REST
Dumbbell reverse lunge	4 X 8 each leg	1 minute 30 seconds	2 X 15 each leg	45 seconds
Push-ups	4 X 8	1 minute 30 seconds	2 X 15	45 seconds
Dumbbell goblet squat	4 X 10	1 minute 30 seconds	4 X 20	45 seconds
Dumbbell row	4 X 8	1 minute 30 seconds	2 X 15	45 seconds

Squat stretch: Sit in a deep squat and put your palms together and push your elbows into the inside of your knee as you push your knees into your elbow.

Dumbbell goblet squat: Position the dumbbell vertically at your chest. Descend by pushing your hips back and bending the knees simultaneously. Once your thighs are at least parallel with the floor (or as low as you can comfortably go), reverse the movement.

Mountain climber jumps: Start in a top press-up position with your hands flat on the floor and your feet about shoulder-width apart. Then explosively bring your knees to your chest, landing your feet on the floor and jumping back out to the starting position.

Mountain climber: Start in a top press-up position with your hands flat on the floor and your feet about shoulder-width apart. Bring one knee toward your chest and return it to the starting position. Replicate the movement with your other leg and continue alternating legs.

Dumbbell lunges: Stand with dumbbells at your side, palms facing your body. Step forward as far as you can with your one leg, bending your trailing knee so it almost touches the floor. Use the heel of your stepping foot to push your upper body back to the starting position, then repeat with the opposite leg.

Push-up with shoulder tap: Start in a top press-up position with your hands flat on the floor and your feet about shoulder-width apart. Lower your chest toward the ground by bending your elbows and pointing them behind you. Push back up to straighten your arms into top press-up position, then lift you right hand to tap your left shoulder at the top. Repeat with the opposite arm tapping.

Dumbbell squat press: Stand with your feet shoulder-width apart, hold dumbbells next to your shoulders. Descend by pushing your hips back and bending the knees simultaneously. Once your thighs are at least parallel with the floor (or as low as you can comfortably go) push your body up from the squat as you press the dumbbells over your head. Your biceps should be by your ears. Lower the weights and repeat.

Jumping jacks: Standing with feet together and your arms to your side, jumping to a position with the legs spread wide and the hands going overhead, and then returning to a position with the feet together and the arms at the sides.

Dumbbell step up: Start by standing in front of a box or bench around knee height, holding dumbbells at your sides with arms straight. Place one foot firmly on the box or bench, then drive through that foot to lift your body up until that leg is straight and your opposite foot is elevated. Step down and repeat with the opposite leg.

Side plank: Lie on your side, legs extended in a straight line from hip to feet. The elbow of your other arm is directly under your shoulder. Make sure your head is directly in line with your spine. Engage your abdominal muscles, drawing your navel toward your spine. Lift your hips and knees from the floor. Your torso is straight in line with no drooping or bending. Hold this position.

Dumbbell shoulder press: Holding the dumbbells by your shoulders, extend through your elbows to press the weights above your head and slowly return to the starting position.

Jump squat: Stand tall with your feet hip-width apart. Descend by pushing your hips back and bending the knees simultaneously. Once your thighs are at least parallel with the floor (or as low as you can comfortably go), push your feet into the ground to explode off the floor and jump as high as you can. Bend your knees when you land, and then immediately drop back down into a squat.

Leg raise: Lie on your back with legs straight and together. With your legs together and as straight as you can, lift them all the way up toward the ceiling until your butt comes off the floor. Slowly lower your legs back down till they almost touch the floor. Raise your legs back up.

Dumbbell renegade: With dumbbells or kettlebells, get into a press-up position with a weight in each hand. Raise one of the weights, supporting yourself on the other arm. Pull the weight upward until your elbow is slightly higher than your torso, then lower it back to the ground. Repeat with the opposite arm.

Jump rope: Hold the rope, standing in front of it while keeping your hands at hip level. Rotate your wrists, pulling the rope underneath to swing the rope and jump. You can jump with both feet at the same time, one foot at a time, or alternating between feet.

Push-up: Start in a top press-up position with your hands flat on the floor and your feet about shoulder-width apart, placing your hands slightly wider than your shoulders. Lower your body until your chest nearly touches the floor, then push yourself back up. Repeat.

REFERENCES

Chapter One

de Martel C, Georges D, Bray F, Ferlay J, Clifford GM. Global burden of cancer attributable to infections in 2018: a worldwide incidence analysis. *Lancet Glob Health.* 2020; 8(2):e180–e190. doi:10.1016/S2214-109X(19)30488-7.

Del Pup L, Peccatori FA, Levi-Setti PE, Codacci-Pisanelli G, Patrizio P. Risk of cancer after assisted reproduction: a review of the available evidences and guidance to fertility counselors. *Eur Rev Med Pharmacol Sci.* 2018; 22(22):8042–8059. doi:10.26355/eurrev_201811_16434.

Friedman GD, Udaltsova N, Chan J, Quesenberry CP Jr, Habel LA. Screening pharmaceuticals for possible carcinogenic effects: initial positive results for drugs not previously screened. *Cancer Causes Control.* 2009; 20(10):1821–1835. doi:10.1007/s10552-009-9375-2.

Giat E, Ehrenfeld M, Shoenfeld Y. Cancer and autoimmune diseases. *Autoimmun Rev.* 2017; 16(10):1049–1057. doi:10.1016/j.autrev.2017.07.022.

Goto A, Yamaji T, Sawada N, et al. Diabetes and cancer risk: A Mendelian randomization study. *Int J Cancer.* 2020; 146(3):712–719. doi:10.1002/ijc.32310.

Iezzoni LI, Rao SR, Agaronnik ND, El-Jawahri A. Cross-sectional analysis of the associations between four common cancers and disability. *J Natl Compr Canc Netw.* 2020; 18:1031–1044. doi:10.6004/jnccn.2020.7551.

Jung JM, Lee KH, Kim YJ, et al. Assessment of overall and specific cancer risks in patients with hidradenitis suppurativa [published online ahead of print, 2020 May 27]. *JAMA Dermatol.* 2020; 156(8):1–10. doi:10.1001/jamadermatol.2020.1422.

Lewis-Mikhael AM, Bueno-Cavanillas A, Ofir Giron T, Olmedo-Requena R, Delgado-Rodríguez M, Jiménez-Moleón JJ. Occupational exposure to pesticides and prostate cancer: a systematic review and meta-analysis [published correction appears in *Occup Environ Med.* 2017 Sep;74(9):699]. *Occup Environ Med.* 2016; 73(2):134–144. doi:10.1136/oemed-2014-102692.

Ligibel JA, Jones LW, Brewster AM, et al. Oncologists' attitudes and practice of addressing diet, physical activity, and weight management with patients with cancer: findings of an ASCO survey of the oncology workforce. *J Oncol Pract.* 2019 Jun;15(6):e520–e528. doi: 10.1200/JOP.19.00124. Epub 2019 May 16. PMID: 31095436; PMCID: PMC6827390.

Loomis D, Guha N, Hall AL, Straif K. Identifying occupational carcinogens: an update from the IARC Monographs. *Occup Environ Med.* 2018; 75(8):593–603. doi:10.1136/oemed-2017-104944.

Marant Micallef C, Shield KD, Baldi I, et al. Occupational exposures and cancer: a review of agents and relative risk estimates. *Occup Environ Med.* 2018; 75(8):604–614. doi:10.1136/oemed-2017-104858.

Memon A, Rogers I, Paudyal P, Sundin J. Dental x-rays and the risk of thyroid cancer and meningioma: a systematic review and meta-analysis of current epidemiological evidence. *Thyroid.* 2019 Nov; 29(11):1572–1593. doi: 10.1089/thy.2019.0105. Epub 2019 Oct 14. PMID: 31502516.

Michaud DS, Lu J, Peacock-Villada AY, et al. Periodontal disease assessed using clinical dental measurements and cancer risk in the ARIC study. *J Natl Cancer Inst.* 2018; 110(8):843–854. doi:10.1093/jnci/djx278.

Mostafalou S, Abdollahi M. Pesticides: an update of human exposure and toxicity. *Arch Toxicol.* 2017; 91(2):549–599. doi:10.1007/s00204-016-1849-x.

Muthukrishnan A, Warnakulasuriya S. Oral health consequences of smokeless tobacco use. *Indian J Med Res.* 2018; 148(1):35–40. doi:10.4103/ijmr.IJMR_1793_17.

Patel S, Sangeeta S. Pesticides as the drivers of neuropsychotic diseases, cancers, and teratogenicity among agro-workers as well as general public. *Environ Sci Pollut Res Int.* 2019; 26(1):91-100. doi:10.1007/s11356-018-3642-2.

Pedersen SA, Gaist D, Schmidt SAJ, Hölmich LR, Friis S, Pottegård A. Hydrochlorothiazide use and risk of nonmelanoma skin cancer: A nationwide case-control study from Denmark. *J Am Acad Dermatol.* 2018; 78(4):673–681.e9. doi:10.1016/j.jaad.2017.11.042.

Pischon T, Nimptsch K. Obesity and risk of cancer: an introductory overview. *Recent Results Cancer Res.* 2016; 208:1–15. doi:10.1007/978-3 -319-42542-9_1.

Rothenberger NJ, Somasundaram A, Stabile LP. The role of the estrogen pathway in the tumor microenvironment. *Int J Mol Sci.* 2018; 19(2):611. Published 2018 Feb 19. doi:10.3390/ijms19020611.

Sakellariou D, Rotarou ES. Cancer disparities for people with disabilities: bridging the gap. *J Natl Compr Canc Netw.* 2020; 18(8):1144– 1146. doi:10.6004/jnccn.2020.7614.

Sample A, He YY. Mechanisms and prevention of UV-induced melanoma. *Photodermatol Photoimmunol Photomed.* 2018; 34(1):13–24. doi:10.1111/phpp.12329.

Turati F, Galeone C, Augustin LSA, La Vecchia C. Glycemic index, glycemic load and cancer risk: an updated meta-analysis. *Nutrients.* 2019; 11(10):2342. Published 2019 Oct 2. doi:10.3390/nu11102342.

Wang W, Xu D, Wang B, et al. Increased risk of cancer in relation to gout: a review of three prospective cohort studies with 50,358 subjects. *Mediators Inflamm.* 2015; 2015:680853. doi:10.1155/2015/680853.

Wojciechowska J, Krajewski W, Bolanowski M, Kręcicki T, Zatoński T. Diabetes and cancer: a review of current knowledge. *Exp Clin Endocrinol Diabetes.* 2016; 124(5):263–275. doi:10.1055/s-0042-100910.

Chapter Two

Bravo-Iñiguez CE, Fox SW, De Leon LE, Tarascio JN, Jaklitsch MT, Jacobson FL. Cumulative nonsmoking risk factors increase the probability of developing lung cancer. *J Thorac Cardiovasc Surg.* 2019; 158(4):1248–1254.e1. doi:10.1016/j.jtcvs.2019.04.098.

Cho YA, Lee J, Oh JH, et al. Genetic risk score, combined lifestyle factors and risk of colorectal cancer. *Cancer Res Treat.* 2019; 51(3):1033– 1040. doi:10.4143/crt.2018.447.

Gandaglia G, van den Bergh RCN, Tilki D, et al. How can we expand active surveillance criteria in patients with low- and intermediate-risk prostate cancer without increasing the risk of misclassification? Development of a novel risk calculator. *BJU Int.* 2018; 122(5):823–830. doi:10.1111/bju.14391.

Olsen CM, Pandeya N, Thompson BS, et al. Risk stratification for melanoma: models derived and validated in a purpose-designed prospective cohort. *J Natl Cancer Inst.* 2018; 110(10):1075–1083. doi:10.1093/jnci/djy023.

Stark GF, Hart GR, Nartowt BJ, Deng J. Predicting breast cancer risk using personal health data and machine learning models. *PLoS One.* 2019; 14(12):e0226765. Published 2019 Dec 27. doi:10.1371/journal .pone.0226765.

Tracey EH, Vij A. Updates in melanoma. *Dermatol Clin.* 2019; 37(1): 73–82. doi:10.1016/j.det.2018.08.003.

Chapter Three

Agurs-Collins T, Ferrer R, Ottenbacher A, Waters EA, O'Connell ME, Hamilton JG. Public awareness of direct-to-consumer genetic tests: findings from the 2013 U.S. Health Information National Trends Survey. *J Cancer Educ.* 2015; 30(4):799–807. doi:10.1007/s13187-014-0784-x.

Covolo L, Rubinelli S, Ceretti E, Gelatti U. Internet-based direct-to-consumer genetic testing: a systematic review. *J Med Internet Res.* 2015; 17(12):e279. Published 2015 Dec 14. doi:10.2196/jmir.4378.

Cragun D, Weidner A, Kechik J, Pal T. Genetic testing across young Hispanic and non-Hispanic white breast cancer survivors: facilitators, barriers, and awareness of the Genetic Information Nondiscrimination Act. *Genet Test Mol Biomarkers.* 2019; 23(2):75–83. doi:10.1089/gtmb .2018.0253.

Hooker GW, Clemens KR, Quillin J, et al. Cancer genetic counseling and testing in an era of rapid change. *J Genet Couns.* 2017; 26(6):1244–1253. doi:10.1007/s10897-017-0099-2.

Hooker SE Jr, Woods-Burnham L, Bathina M, et al. Genetic ancestry analysis reveals misclassification of commonly used cancer cell lines. *Cancer Epidemiol Biomarkers Prev.* 2019; 28(6):1003–1009. doi:10.1158 /1055-9965.EPI-18-1132.

Kirkpatrick BE, Rashkin MD. Ancestry testing and the practice of genetic counseling. *J Genet Couns.* 2017; 26(1):6–20. doi:10.1007 /s10897-016-0014-2.

Marzulla T, Roberts JS, DeVries R, Koeller DR, Green RC, Uhlmann WR. Genetic counseling following direct-to-consumer genetic testing: consumer perspectives [published online ahead of print, 2020 Jul 9]. *J Genet Couns.* 2020; 10.1002/jgc4.1309. doi:10.1002/jgc4.1309.

Reed EK, Edelman EA. Direct-to-consumer genetic testing for breast cancer risk. *J Am Assoc Nurse Pract.* 2018; 30(10):548–550. doi:10.1097/JXX.0000000000000146.

Chapter Four

Abbasi J, Devries S. Training physicians about nutrition. *JAMA.* 2018; 319(17):1751–1752. doi:10.1001/jama.2018.1070.

Chiesa Fuxench ZC, Shin DB, Ogdie Beatty A, Gelfand JM. The risk of cancer in patients with psoriasis: a population-based cohort study in the Health Improvement Network. *JAMA Dermatol.* 2016; 152(3):282–290. doi:10.1001/jamadermatol.2015.4847.

Chou R, Dana T, Fu R, et al. Screening for hepatitis C virus infection in adolescents and adults: updated evidence report and systematic review for the US Preventive Services Task Force [published online ahead of print, 2020 Mar 2]. *JAMA.* 2020; 10.1001/jama.2019.20788. doi:10.1001/jama.2019.20788.

Elinav E, Garrett WS, Trinchieri G, Wargo J. The cancer microbiome. *Nat Rev Cancer.* 2019 Jul; 19(7):371–376. doi: 10.1038/s41568-019-0155-3. Epub 2019 Jun 11. PMID: 31186547; PMCID: PMC6700740.

Fontham ETH, Wolf A, Church TR, et al. Cervical cancer screening for individuals at average risk: 2020 guideline update from the American Cancer Society. *CA Cancer J Clin.* 2020; 70(5):321–346. Published 2020 Jul 30. doi.org/10.3322/caac.21628.

García-Albéniz X, Hernán MA, Logan RW, Price M, Armstrong K, Hsu J. Continuation of annual screening mammography and breast cancer mortality in women older than 70 years. *Ann Intern Med.* 2020; 172(6): 381–389. doi:10.7326/M18-1199.

Henderson JT, Webber EM, Sawaya GF. Screening for ovarian cancer: updated evidence report and systematic review for the US Preventive Services Task Force. *JAMA.* 2018; 319(6):595–606. doi:10.1001/jama.2017.21421.

Lin JS, Bowles EJA, Williams SB, Morrison CC. Screening for thyroid cancer: updated evidence report and systematic review for the US

Preventive Services Task Force. *JAMA.* 2017;317(18):1888–1903. doi: 10.1001/jama.2017.0562.

Menon U, Karpinskyj C, Gentry-Maharaj A. Ovarian cancer prevention and screening. *Obstet Gynecol.* 2018; 131(5):909–927. doi:10.1097/AOG .0000000000002580.

Nattinger AB, Mitchell JL. Breast cancer screening and prevention. *Ann Intern Med.* 2016; 164(11):ITC81-ITC96. doi:10.7326/AITC201606070.

Niell BL, Freer PE, Weinfurtner RJ, Arleo EK, Drukteinis JS. Screening for breast cancer. *Radiol Clin North Am.* 2017; 55(6):1145–1162. doi:10 .1016/j.rcl.2017.06.004.

Schünemann HJ, Lerda D, Quinn C, et al. Breast cancer screening and diagnosis: a synopsis of the European breast guidelines. *Ann Intern Med.* 2020; 172(1):46–56. doi:10.7326/M19-2125.

Smith RA, Andrews KS, Brooks D, et al. Cancer screening in the United States, 2019: A review of current American Cancer Society guidelines and current issues in cancer screening. *CA Cancer J Clin.* 2019; 69(3):184–210. doi:10.3322/caac.21557.

Chapter Five

Alexander DD, Weed DL, Miller PE, Mohamed MA. Red meat and colorectal cancer: a quantitative update on the state of the epidemiologic science. *J Am Coll Nutr.* 2015; 34(6):521–543. doi:10.108 0/07315724.2014.992553.

Alicandro G, Tavani A, La Vecchia C. Coffee and cancer risk: a summary overview. *Eur J Cancer Prev.* 2017; 26(5):424–432. doi:10.1097/CEJ .0000000000000341.

Flood DM, Weiss NS, Cook LS, Emerson JC, Schwartz SM, Potter JD. Colorectal cancer incidence in Asian migrants to the United States and their descendants. *Cancer Causes Control.* 2000; 11(5):403–411. doi:10 .1023/a:1008955722425.

Górska A, Przystupski D, Niemczura MJ, Kulbacka J. Probiotic bacteria: a promising tool in cancer prevention and therapy. *Curr Microbiol.* 2019; 76(8):939–949. doi:10.1007/s00284-019-01679-8.

Hydes TJ, Burton R, Inskip H, Bellis MA, Sheron N. A comparison of gender-linked population cancer risks between alcohol and tobacco: how many cigarettes are there in a bottle of wine? *BMC Public Health.*

2019 Mar 28; 19(1):316. doi: 10.1186/s12889-019-6576-9. PMID: 30917803; PMCID: PMC6437970.

Kim J, Park MK, Li WQ, Qureshi AA, Cho E. Association of vitamin A intake with cutaneous squamous cell carcinoma risk in the United States [published online ahead of print, 2019 Jul 31]. *JAMA Dermatol.* 2019; 155(11):1260–1268. doi:10.1001/jamadermatol.2019.1937.

Maskarinec G, Noh JJ. The effect of migration on cancer incidence among Japanese in Hawaii. *Ethn Dis.* 2004; 14(3):431–439.

Messina M. Impact of soy foods on the development of breast cancer and the prognosis of breast cancer patients. *Forsch Komplementmed.* 2016; 23(2):75–80. doi: 10.1159/000444735. Epub 2016 Apr 12. PMID: 27161216.

Mozaffarian D, Hao T, Rimm EB, Willett WC, Hu FB. Changes in diet and lifestyle and long-term weight gain in women and men. *N Engl J Med.* 2011; 364(25):2392–2404. doi:10.1056/NEJMoa1014296.

Pereira MA. Sugar-sweetened and artificially-sweetened beverages in relation to obesity risk. *Adv Nutr.* 2014; 5(6):797–808. Published 2014 Nov 14. doi:10.3945/an.114.007062.

Rowles JL 3rd, Ranard KM, Smith JW, An R, Erdman JW Jr. Increased dietary and circulating lycopene are associated with reduced prostate cancer risk: a systematic review and meta-analysis. *Prostate Cancer Prostatic Dis.* 2017; 20(4):361–377. doi:10.1038/pcan.2017.25.

Ruanpeng D, Thongprayoon C, Cheungpasitporn W, Harindhanavudhi T. Sugar and artificially sweetened beverages linked to obesity: a systematic review and meta-analysis. *QJM.* 2017; 110(8):513–520. doi:10.1093/qjmed/hcx068.

Salehi M, Moradi-Lakeh M, Salehi MH, Nojomi M, Kolahdooz F. Meat, fish, and esophageal cancer risk: a systematic review and dose-response meta-analysis. *Nutr Rev.* 2013; 71(5):257–267. doi:10.1111/nure.12028.

Schwingshackl L, Hoffmann G, Buijsse B, et al. Dietary supplements and risk of cause-specific death, cardiovascular disease, and cancer: a protocol for a systematic review and network meta-analysis of primary prevention trials. *Syst Rev.* 2015; 4:34. Published 2015 Mar 26. doi:10.1186/s13643-015-0029-z.

Srour B, Fezeu LK, Kesse-Guyot E, et al. Ultraprocessed food consumption and risk of type 2 diabetes among participants of the NutriNet-Santé prospective cohort. *JAMA Intern Med.* 2020; 180(2): 283–291. doi:10.1001/jamainternmed.2019.5942.

Thiébaut AC, Jiao L, Silverman DT, et al. Dietary fatty acids and pancreatic cancer in the NIH-AARP diet and health study. *J Natl Cancer Inst.* 2009; 101(14):1001–1011. doi:10.1093/jnci/djp168.

Yang W, Ma Y, Liu Y, et al. Association of intake of whole grains and dietary fiber with risk of hepatocellular carcinoma in US adults. *JAMA Oncol.* 2019; 5(6):879–886. doi:10.1001/jamaoncol.2018.7159.

Zhao Z, Yin Z, Zhao Q. Red and processed meat consumption and gastric cancer risk: a systematic review and meta-analysis. *Oncotarget.* 2017; 8(18):30563–30575. doi:10.18632/oncotarget.15699.

Chapter Six

Cormie P, Zopf EM, Zhang X, Schmitz KH. The impact of exercise on cancer mortality, recurrence, and treatment-related adverse effects. *Epidemiol Rev.* 2017; 39(1):71–92. doi:10.1093/epirev/mxx007.

Cramer H, Lauche R, Klose P, Lange S, Langhorst J, Dobos GJ. Yoga for improving health-related quality of life, mental health, and cancer-related symptoms in women diagnosed with breast cancer. *Cochrane Database Syst Rev.* 2017 Jan 3; 1(1):CD010802. doi: 10.1002/14651858 .CD010802.pub2. PMID: 28045199; PMCID: PMC6465041.

Dimitrov S, Hulteng E, Hong S. Inflammation and exercise: Inhibition of monocytic intracellular TNF production by acute exercise via β2-adrenergic activation. *Brain Behav Immun.* 2017; 61:60–68. doi:10.1016/j.bbi.2016.12.017.

Hojman P, Gehl J, Christensen JF, Pedersen BK. Molecular mechanisms linking exercise to cancer prevention and treatment. *Cell Metab.* 2018; 27(1):10–21. doi:10.1016/j.cmet.2017.09.015.

Idorn M, Hojman P. Exercise-dependent regulation of NK cells in cancer protection. *Trends Mol Med.* 2016; 22(7):565–577. doi:10.1016 /j.molmed.2016.05.007.

Kraschnewski JL, Schmitz KH. Exercise in the prevention and treatment of breast cancer: what clinicians need to tell their patients. *Curr Sports Med Rep.* 2017; 16(4):263–267. doi:10.1249/JSR .0000000000000388.

McGee SL, Hargreaves M. Epigenetics and exercise. *Trends Endocrinol Metab.* 2019; 30(9):636–645. doi:10.1016/j.tem.2019.06.002.

Rezapour S, Shiravand M, Mardani M. Epigenetic changes due to physical activity. *Biotechnol Appl Biochem.* 2018; 65(6):761–767. doi:10 .1002/bab.1689.

Scmitz K, Campbell A, Stuiver M, et al. Exercise is medicine in oncology: engaging clinicians to help patients move through cancer. *CA Cancer J Clin.* 2019; 69:468–484.

Shaw DM, Merien F, Braakhuis A, Dulson D. T-cells and their cytokine production: The anti-inflammatory and immunosuppressive effects of strenuous exercise. *Cytokine.* 2018; 104:136–142. doi:10.1016/j.cyto .2017.10.001.

Simioni C, Zauli G, Martelli AM, et al. Oxidative stress: role of physical exercise and antioxidant nutraceuticals in adulthood and aging. *Oncotarget.* 2018; 9(24):17181–17198. Published 2018 Mar 30. doi:10 .18632/oncotarget.24729.

Stamatakis E, Lee IM, Bennie J, et al. Does strength-promoting exercise confer unique health benefits? A pooled analysis of data on 11 population cohorts with all-cause, cancer, and cardiovascular mortality endpoints. *Am J Epidemiol.* 2018; 187(5):1102–1112. doi:10.1093/aje /kwx345.

Chapter Seven

Bahri N, Fathi Najafi T, Homaei Shandiz F, Tohidinik HR, Khajavi A. The relation between stressful life events and breast cancer: a systematic review and meta-analysis of cohort studies. *Breast Cancer Res Treat.* 2019; 176(1):53–61. doi:10.1007/s10549-019-05231-x.

Boehm JK, Chen Y, Koga H, Mathur MB, Vie LL, Kubzansky LD. Is optimism associated with healthier cardiovascular-related behavior? Meta-Analyses of 3 Health Behaviors. *Circ Res.* 2018 Apr 13; 122(8): 1119–1134. doi: 10.1161/CIRCRESAHA.117.310828. PMID: 29650630.

Boehm JK, Williams DR, Rimm EB, Ryff C, Kubzansky LD. Association between optimism and serum antioxidants in the midlife in the United States study. *Psychosom Med.* 2013 Jan; 75(1):2–10. doi: 10.1097/PSY .0b013e31827c08a9. Epub 2012 Dec 20. PMID: 23257932; PMCID: PMC3539819.

Cole SW. Social regulation of human gene expression: mechanisms and implications for public health. *Am J Public Health.* 2013; 103 Suppl 1(Suppl 1):S84–S92. doi:10.2105/AJPH.2012.301183.

Goessl VC, Curtiss JE, Hofmann SG. The effect of heart rate variability biofeedback training on stress and anxiety: a meta-analysis. *Psychol Med.* 2017 Nov; 47(15):2578–2586. doi: 10.1017/S0033291717001003. Epub 2017 May 8. PMID: 28478782.

Gross AL, Gallo JJ, Eaton WW. Depression and cancer risk: 24 years of follow-up of the Baltimore Epidemiologic Catchment Area sample. *Cancer Causes Control.* 2010; 21(2):191–199. doi:10.1007/s10552-009 -9449-1.

Jia Y, Li F, Liu YF, Zhao JP, Leng MM, Chen L. Depression and cancer risk: a systematic review and meta-analysis. *Public Health.* 2017; 149:138– 148. doi:10.1016/j.puhe.2017.04.026.

Khoshnood Z, Iranmanesh S, Rayyani M, Dehghan M. Body-mind healing strategies in patients with cancer: a qualitative content analysis. *Asian Pac J Cancer Prev.* 2018 Jun 25; 19(6):1691–1696. doi: 10.22034 /APJCP.2018.19.6.1691. PMID: 29938467; PMCID: PMC6103568.

Ko, A., Kim, K., Sik Son, J. et al. Association of pre-existing depression with all-cause, cancer-related, and noncancer-related mortality among 5-year cancer survivors: a population-based cohort study. *Sci Rep* 9, 18334 (2019). https://doi.org/10.1038/s41598-019-54677-y.

Littrell J. The mind-body connection: not just a theory anymore. *Soc Work Health Care.* 2008; 46(4):17–37. doi: 10.1300/j010v46n04_02. PMID: 18589562.

Mukherjee S. Cancer, our genes, and the anxiety of risk-based medicine. *Health Aff (Millwood).* 2018; 37(5):817–820. doi:10.1377 /hlthaff.2018.0344.

Sztachańska J, Krejtz I, Nezlek JB. Using a gratitude intervention to improve the lives of women with breast cancer: a daily diary study. *Front Psychol.* 2019 Jun 12; 10:1365. doi: 10.3389/fpsyg.2019.01365. PMID: 31249544; PMCID: PMC6582750.

Toussaint L, Barry M, Angus D, Bornfriend L, Markman M. Self-forgiveness is associated with reduced psychological distress in cancer patients and unmatched caregivers: hope and self-blame as mediating mechanisms. *J Psychosoc Oncol.* 2017; 35(5):544–560. doi:10 .1080/07347332.2017.1309615.

Yang T, Qiao Y, Xiang S, Li W, Gan Y, Chen Y. Work stress and the risk of cancer: A meta-analysis of observational studies. *Int J Cancer.* 2019; 144(10):2390–2400. doi:10.1002/ijc.31955.

Chapter Eight

Bjorness TE, Greene RW. Adenosine and sleep. *Curr Neuropharmacol.* 2009; 7(3):238–245. doi:10.2174/157015909789152182.

Chen Y, Tan F, Wei L, et al. Sleep duration and the risk of cancer: a systematic review and meta-analysis including dose-response relationship. *BMC Cancer.* 2018; 18(1):1149. Published 2018 Nov 21. doi:10.1186/s12885-018-5025-y.

Cribbet MR, Carlisle M, Cawthon RM. Cellular aging and restorative processes: subjective sleep quality and duration moderate the association between age and telomere length in a sample of middle-aged and older adults. *Sleep.* 2014; 37(1). doi:org/10.5665 /sleep.3308.

Daniels RD, Kibale TL, Yiin JH, et al. Mortality and cancer incidence in a pooled cohort of firefighters form San Francisco, Chicago and Philadelphia. *Occupational and Environmental Medicine* 71 (6): 388–397.

Foster RG. Sleep, circadian rhythms, and health. *Interface Focus.* 2020; 10(3):20190098. doi:10.1098/rsfs.2019.0098.

Gan Y, Li L, Zhang L, et al. Association between shift work and risk of prostate cancer: a systematic review and meta-analysis of observational studies. *Carcinogenesis.* 2018; 39(2):87–97. doi:10.1093/carcin/bgx129.

Lu C, Sun H, Huang J, et al. Long-term sleep duration as a risk factor for breast cancer: evidence from a systematic review and dose-response meta-analysis. *Biomed Res Int.* 2017; 2017:4845059. doi:10.1155/2017 /4845059

Monti JM. Serotonin control of sleep-wake behavior. *Sleep Med Rev.* 2011; 15(4):269-81. doi: 10.1016/j.smrv.2010.11.003. Epub 2011 Apr 2. PMID: 21459634.

Rivera AS, Akanbi M, O'Dwyer LC, McHugh M. Shift work and long work hours and their association with chronic health conditions: A systematic review of systematic reviews with meta-analyses. *PLoS One.* 2020; 15(4):e0231037. Published 2020 Apr 2. doi:10.1371/journal .pone.0231037.

Wang P, Ren FM, Lin Y, et al. Night-shift work, sleep duration, daytime napping, and breast cancer risk. *Sleep Med.* 2015; 16(4):462–468. doi:10 .1016/j.sleep.2014.11.017.

Zhao H, Yin JY, Yang WS, et al. Sleep duration and cancer risk: a systematic review and meta-analysis of prospective studies. *Asian Pac J Cancer Prev.* 2013; 14(12):7509–7515. doi:10.7314/apjcp.2013.14.12.7509.

Chapter Nine

Bowen WS, Svrivastava AK, Batra L, Barsoumian H, Shirwan H. Current challenges for cancer vaccine adjuvant development. *Expert Rev Vaccines.* 2018 Mar; 17(3):207–215. doi: 10.1080/14760584.2018.1434000. Epub 2018 Feb 8. PMID: 29372660; PMCID: PMC6093214.

Brouwer AF, Delinger RL, Eisenberg MC, et al. HPV vaccination has not increased sexual activity or accelerated sexual debut in a college-aged cohort of men and women. *BMC Public Health.* 2019 Jun 25; 19(1):821. doi: 10.1186/s12889-019-7134-1. PMID: 31238911; PMCID: PMC6593582.

Haber P, Moro PL, Ng C, et al. Safety of currently licensed hepatitis B surface antigen vaccines in the United States, Vaccine Adverse Event Reporting System (VAERS), 2005–2015. *Vaccine.* 2018 Jan 25; 36(4):559–564. doi: 10.1016/j.vaccine.2017.11.079. Epub 2017 Dec 11. PMID: 29241647.

Handy CE, Antonarakis ES. Sipuleucel-T for the treatment of prostate cancer: novel insights and future directions. *Future Oncol.* 2018 Apr; 14(10):907–917. doi: 10.2217/fon-2017-0531. Epub 2017 Dec 20. PMID: 29260582; PMCID: PMC5925432.

Holman DM, Benard V, Roland KB, Watson M, Liddon N, Stokley S. Barriers to human papillomavirus vaccination among US adolescents: a systematic review of the literature. *JAMA Pediatr.* 2014 Jan; 168(1):76–82. doi: 10.1001/jamapediatrics.2013.2752. PMID: 24276343; PMCID: PMC4538997.

Johnson DB, Puzanov I, Kelley MC. Talimogene laherparepvec (T-VEC) for the treatment of advanced melanoma. *Immunotherapy.* 2015; 7(6):611–9. doi: 10.2217/imt.15.35. Epub 2015 Jun 22. PMID: 26098919; PMCID: PMC4519012.

Morales A. BCG: A throwback from the stone age of vaccines opened the path for bladder cancer immunotherapy. *Can J Urol.* 2017 Jun; 24(3):8788–8793. PMID: 28646932.

Pettenati C, Ingersoll MA. Mechanisms of BCG immunotherapy and its outlook for bladder cancer. *Nat Rev Urol.* 2018 Oct; 15(10):615–625. doi: 10.1038/s41585-018-0055-4. PMID: 29991725.

Tau N, Yahav D, Shepshelovich D. Postmarketing Safety of Vaccines Approved by the U.S. Food and Drug Administration: a cohort study. *Ann Intern Med.* 2020 Sep 15; 173(6):445–449. doi: 10.7326/M20-2726. Epub 2020 Jul 28. PMID: 32716700.

INDEX

ABOUT THE AUTHOR

JOHN WHYTE, MD, MPH, is a popular physician and writer who has been communicating to the public about health issues for nearly two decades.

In his role as chief medical officer of WebMD, Dr. Whyte leads efforts to develop and expand strategic partnerships that create meaningful change around important and timely public health issues. Before joining WebMD, Whyte served as the director of professional affairs and stakeholder engagement at the Center for Drug Evaluation and Research at the US Food and Drug Administration. Dr. Whyte worked with health care professionals, patients, and patient advocates, providing them with a focal point for advocacy, enhanced two-way communication, and collaboration, assisting them in navigating the FDA on issues concerning drug development, review, and drug safety. He also developed numerous initiatives to address diversity in clinical trials.

Dr. Whyte worked for nearly a decade as the chief medical expert and vice president, health and medical education, at Discovery Channel, the leading nonfiction television network. In this role, he developed, designed, and delivered educational programming that appealed to medical and lay audiences. This included television shows and on-line content that won more than fifty awards, including numerous Tellys, CINE Golden Eagles, and Freddies.

Whyte is a board-certified internist. He completed an internal medicine residency at Duke University Medical Center and earned a master of public health in health policy and management at Harvard University School of Public Health. Before arriving in Washington, DC, he was a health services research fellow at Stanford and attending physician in the department of medicine.